My Rose

My Rose

An African American Mother's Story of AIDS

GENEVA E. BELL

United Church Press

Cleveland, Ohio

United Church Press, Cleveland, Ohio 44115
© 1997 by Geneva E. Bell

Printed in the United States of America on acid-free paper

02 01 00 99 98   5 4 3 2

Library of Congress Cataloging-in-Publication Data

    Bell, Geneva E., 1929–
       My rose : an African American mother's story of AIDS /
    Geneva E. Bell.
           p.   cm.
     ISBN 0-8298-1160-5 (alk. paper)
     1. Bell, Jeffery, 1959–1992—Health. 2. AIDS (Disease)—
Patients—United States—Biography. 3. Afro-American
gays—Biography. 4. Bell, Geneva E., 1929– . 5. Mothers—
United States—Biography. I. Title.
RC607.A26B444   1997
362.1'969792'0092—dc21   97-3419
  [B]   CIP

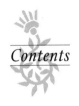

Contents

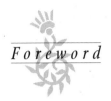

Foreword

 he story of Jeffery Bell and his family is a story that needs to be told all over North America and especially all over black America. The response of Jeff's church, the reaction of Jeff's family, and the reaffirmation of Jeff's faith are both tragic and triumphant; and they need to be studied by persons of faith everywhere who are confronted with the reality of HIV/AIDS.

Jeffery was an absolutely delightful person. He was the kind of man all pastors wish to have in their congregations. He was dedicated. He was sincere. He was authentic. He was transparent. And he was real.

Jeff came to me before joining Trinity UCC to talk to me about his sexual orientation, and the problems that this orientation had caused him (and his family) prior to his decision to become a part of our church family. He felt cheated and trapped. He had no choice as to the way God had created him. He had no choice as to the way he had been for as long as he could remember. He was born with a same-sex orientation, and he did not understand that or appreciate it. He wanted to know why God had done that to him.

After our initial series of conversations, Jeff joined our church and became one of our most active, sincere, and dedicated members. He threw himself into the life and work of the congregation, and he made dozens of friends in the process.

When Jeff became HIV-positive he did not share that fact

with me, and I was at a loss in terms of understanding why! After all, we had shared as pastor and parishioner his sexual orientation. We had shared the problems his orientation had caused him in his family, in the service, in the fraternity, and in the congregation. We had shared the pain he suffered and the stereotypes he endured. Yet, when it came to the most important sharing, Jeff initially chose to keep that to himself.

In the pages that follow, Geneva Bell shares her experiences as a mother, a Christian, and a deacon. You need to read her words carefully and prayerfully. Much of the pain she experienced was inflicted by well-meaning Christians whose closed minds and prejudicial opinions hurt far more than words can describe. Here in these few lines I want to give you the perspective of a pastor who tried (and still tries) to do ministry under some incredibly unbelievable circumstances.

I got word that Jeffery was in the hospital and I went to pay him what I thought was a normal pastoral visit. When I got to his room, I was met with the "Mask and Gown Required" signs; in 90 percent of the cases where I had seen that sign, the patients had full-blown AIDS or were HIV-positive. With thousands of questions running through my mind, I put on my gown and my mask, and went to spend a few moments with my friend, my congregation member, and my fraternity brother.

We talked about much of nothing for a few moments. He had a Saturday afternoon college football game on and we watched for about ten minutes—"oohing and ahhing" over fantastic plays and spectacular runs. Before reading Scripture and having prayer, I asked Jeff why he was there, and I asked him specifically about the mask and gown requirement. Jeff assured me it was hepatitis and that he was highly susceptible to infections from the outside—especially with it being the Chicago cold and flu season.

I almost believed him, but something kept nagging me, and I couldn't just "let it go" at what Jeff was telling me. The next day at church following our second service, I approached one of the men in our congregation who is gay and who was a close friend of Jeff's. I asked him, "What is going on with Jeffery Bell?" Reading the look on my face, he assured me that it was definitely not HIV or AIDS.

"Oh no, Rev," he protested. "I would tell you if that were the case, but it's just some rare form of hepatitis." I didn't know it then, but the pain, the shock, and the reality of what Jeff was facing caused him to withhold the truth from even his closest friends.

I took what his friend said at face value, and I believed that for about a week. But then, however, when Jeffery was still sick, I called one of the staff chaplains at the hospital, and within a matter of seconds he answered me with words that still haunt me to this day. He said, "Pastor Wright, your member has full-blown AIDS."

I sat there numb for a few moments, not knowing what to say or do. Jeff did not want to share that truth with me. He had not even shared it with his close friends at church, and I knew he hadn't shared it with most of his family. I was trapped as a pastor—caught between the proverbial devil and the deep blue sea. I had some crucial knowledge, some vital knowledge, some life-changing knowledge, and the people I needed to talk with about that knowledge were cut off from me either by choice or by the fact that they simply did not know.

After a few weeks, I took a deep breath, prayed a fervent prayer, and confronted Jeffery face to face. We cried together. We laughed together. We prayed together. Then we began to talk about practical and personal matters. I asked him whether he had ever talked to either his mother or his sister who lived in Chicago about his sexuality. He assured me that he had not. I asked him when he planned to do that, and he assured me that he could not.

I talked to him about his mother's love for him—unconditional love—and begged him to go to her and talk with her heart to heart and son to mother. That very afternoon Geneva called my office to ask for an appointment. I just knew the information he had shared with her was more than she could handle and she needed to talk to her pastor about it.

The day of our appointment I took another deep breath, prayed another fervent prayer, and sat down to discuss a Christian perspective on homosexuality. I knew that some of her colleagues (indeed, some of her fellow deacons) and some of her friends were rabidly homophobic, so I thought I would be spending the next couple of hours countering all the "proof texting" that she had had laid on her by those homophobic colleagues and friends. Instead, I got another shock.

After we chatted for a few minutes about little or nothing, she said to me, "Jeffery said you wanted to see me." I looked at her incredulously, shook my head, and asked, "What?"

She said once again, "Jeffery said you wanted to see me. He said you needed to talk to me, so I made this appointment for today. What did you want to talk to me about?"

"You mean Jeffery did not come home and talk to you heart to heart and son to mother last week?" I asked. She said, "No. He came in the house, said you needed to make an appointment with me, and went straight to his room."

"And he hasn't said a word since then?" I asked. "Not about his conversation with you. Just small talk around the house, and my fussing at him about taking his medicine."

In retrospect, I don't know why I was so shocked. For over thirty years this young man had lived with a truth and wrestled with a set of questions for which the church and "Christians" had no answer. How did I think that one or several sessions with me would change the terror with which he had lived for over three decades? Jeffery figured that I could talk to his mother without all the emotional baggage that he would bring to the conversation, so he had arranged the meeting.

We began to talk and Geneva poured out her soul in a climate of refreshing trust and affirmation. Of course she knew her son was gay. No! He had never come to her to talk about what he was feeling, what she was feeling, what people were saying, or what the "church" was teaching. That subject remained an untouched one between the two of them across the years, but being Jeff's mother made it impossible for her *not* to know.

She also knew he was deathly ill. She knew he was taking all kinds of medications, and she knew the medications weren't helping. He was literally dying before her very eyes. She wanted him to talk with her. She wanted to talk to him. But there seemed to be an uncrossable chasm between them that prevented that conversation from ever taking place.

The time we spent together that day turned out to be just the bridge that was needed in order to span that chasm. We spent at least two hours talking about God, talking about homosexuality, talking about HIV/AIDS, talking about assumptions, stereotypes, fears, ignorance, and hatred. We spent the bulk of our time talking about God's love for Jeff, God's love for her, and her love for her son.

We had an absolutely life-changing and liberating conversation. She shared with me how she had thought of leaving the church because of some of the homophobic comments made by her own friends. She shared with me how she had questioned God as to how God could create her son and condemn her son all at the same time. She shared with me all the years of love and care and unanswered questions, and she shared with me the joy of having a pastor who did not bash homosexuals. She went home strengthened, encouraged, and fearful for her child and what he was facing.

As the months wore on and the whispers started circulating around the church as to why Jeffery was losing weight and what the real cause of his illness was, I had to make another pastoral decision. Jeffery not only had a mother and sister in our congregation, he also had a niece and nephew who were both teenagers and both active in the church programs. I wrestled with the question, "How long will it be before they hear something, overhear something, or are confronted with the hearsay, the gossip, and the rumors concerning their uncle?"

I called their mother and asked (rhetorically) if she had talked to them about their favorite uncle, and as I suspected, she had not. I asked how long she planned to delay that conversation, and she tearfully explained to me that she just could not do it. At my request, she brought them by my office after school. I took yet another deep breath, prayed yet another fervent prayer, and plunged into one of the most difficult conversations I have ever had in a quarter of a century of pastoral care.

I talked to the teenagers about sexual orientation and how God created some people different from other people. I talked about the all-important principle of "different not meaning deficient," and got them to understand how crucial it was to grasp that principle. When we were all on the same page, I explained to them that their uncle was homosexual and that he was dying of AIDS.

When the tears started, I wished for a moment that I was in some other profession. Nothing I could say stopped the tears, and nothing their mother said helped either. We prayed. They left and I felt very alone. God showed me in a flash, however, that my feelings were nothing compared to how Jeff must be feeling.

As my colleague Cornel West pointed out, the black church tends to vacillate between denial and denouncement when it comes to the homosexual community in our midst and in our congregations. On the one hand the black church tends to be more conservative than the most rabidly racist "right-winger." On the other hand, the black church ignores a significant segment of its own constituency and misses the opportunity to do ministry on behalf of the one who said "Whatsoever" (to quote Gardner Taylor).

Reading Geneva Bell's story may shake some of us out of the complacency that causes us to miss those opportunities. Even more importantly, reading her story may awaken us to the true meaning of Jesus' words: "Inasmuch as you have done it unto the least of these my little ones, you have done it unto me."

It is certainly my prayer that the latter will be the case.

Rev. Jeremiah A. Wright Jr.
Trinity United Church of Christ
Chicago, Illinois

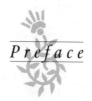

Preface

$\mathscr{T}$here are over a million stories that could have been written by mothers who have lost their children to the dread disease of AIDS (Acquired Immune Deficiency Syndrome). This one is mine. After the death of my son Jeffery, I remained angry. I thought the anger would be toward God, but instead I found myself enraged at people in general, and at my own church members in particular. During Jeff's illness the church was not a safe place for me to talk about my reality. Emotional support and Christian comfort were not available to either one of us. I felt alone. My story was locked within me. My wounded spirit could not be healed.

Shortly after Jeff's death, the deacons group, of which I am a member, held a retreat. To my surprise, my pastor, Rev. Dr. Jeremiah A. Wright Jr., asked me to share with them my painful journey with Jeff. I refused his invitation, telling him that I would not be able to hold back the tears. His response was that God made tears for us to cry. I told this story at the retreat. I shared the painful treatment we received from some members of the congregation and how we had felt abandoned during our ordeal. I told them that I had prayed for some method to help them understand my pain. That time of sharing was the beginning of my healing.

I wrote my pastor, thanking him for asking me to speak,

and telling him that I had kept a journal of my struggle. My plans were to one day write a book. Dr. Wright wrote back: "Not one day, but *now!*" This started another healing process. As this book goes to press, some five years after Jeff's death, God has given me the opportunity to reflect on and see the grace intertwined throughout this distressing situation. That grace continues as both my daughters and myself are now heavily involved in the fight against the ignorance surrounding AIDS.

One of my daughters volunteers at an AIDS hospice in California and my other daughter has been certified by the American Red Cross as an AIDS spokesperson. My local congregation, Trinity United Church of Christ in Chicago, has an outstanding HIV/AIDS ministry with over eighty members to which I belong. Our work is well known around the city as we hold an annual AIDS conference.

I will be forever grateful to my pastor, Rev. Dr. Jeremiah A. Wright Jr., for his encouragement; to my sister in Christ Rev. Dr. Linda H. Hollies for her excellent work in editing this book; to Rev. Paul Sadler, who was Jeff's true friend before and throughout his illness; to Kim Martin Sadler, the editor of United Church Press who believed in this book; and to Rev. James Dawkins, who was always at Jeff's side. There are so many others who helped me along this journey and I would not try to list all their names; they know who they are. I'm forever grateful.

This book is dedicated to all the mothers who have lived or who are now living this story today. I pray for them and hold them in my heart. I also pray that the information shared will cause other congregations to get involved in the growing fight against AIDS.

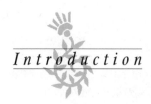

Introduction

It all began with celebrations. From the time he was eighteen years old, my son sent me beautiful roses for every occasion. The rose, a symbol of love and commitment, seemed so appropriate from him, always a tender and thoughtful child. The other children would seek to find new and different trinkets for every event, but Jeff always sent me roses.

I love roses for their fragile beauty, their strong sense of presence, and their lingering loveliness, even as they dry and fade. Roses have come to symbolize my son for me. Even on the day he died, roses were sent to me, on his instructions, by his best friend. I knew there was a significant story waiting to unfurl in the gift of these roses. For even though the petals of the rose are delicate, and their distinct aroma so exquisite, they come from sturdy stock and prickly shrubs. And, with all of their overwhelming beauty, roses have the capacity to cause great pain.

Roses emerge from a family, the Rosaceae family to be exact. They go through growth stages and require much care as they mature and grow. Roses have many particular characteristics such as the bud, the stem, the thorns, the full bloom, the falling petals, and the gradual fade. Yet dried roses are beloved and included in many floral arrangements and artistic designs. So roses never really die. Their usefulness lives on in other forms, even as a fragrant potpourri.

This is the story of my son.

This book is a compilation of things I learned as I traveled with Jeff as he died from AIDS. This story is not mine alone, but a universal one that I participated in and experienced personally. As a Christian and a mother, I continued to seek direction and guidance from my faith. I came to realize that I am Rizpah, the biblical sister who stood for five months guarding the dead bones of her son. At times I was Mary, the mother of Jesus, who stood at the foot of the cross, helpless, but there for her son. Circumstances dictated that part of Ruth emerged in my character as I was determined to follow my loved one into a strange and unfamiliar land. The point came when Esther's resolve became mine, and I declared, "If I perish, I perish, I'm going . . ." Many were the occasions when I felt just like Lot's nameless wife, running wildly, not knowing where we were headed. Yet I am the brave women who walked in the dark to the grave site of Jesus only to be the first to discover that the Rose of Sharon was alive, his fragrance stronger still.

The hopes, dreams, and painful realities of my faith journey and my local church are revealed in the reliving of these memories. I pray that you will both learn and grow from my account, knowing that it is only a story that is told in part. My sincere desire is that you raise awareness in and lend insights to your local congregation as you struggle to do ministry with both my son and myself. We are both in your congregation. We both need your understanding, your acceptance, and your care.

I saw the potential beauty of my rose at the first sight of my newborn son. I watched the slender and tender stem as he encountered life and grew. The years of school, scouts, sports, and Sunday school allowed Jeff to engage in life fully. It seems to me that it was when he was at his most vulnerable stage that his thorns became the most prickly and sharp. But it's the pain of life that draws us closer, and as HIV/AIDS entered our lives, the petals became more poignant and fragrant. Yet I discovered that a rose never dies, for my love for Jeff is stronger than ever. His life was not in vain, and he has much to teach the church about love and beauty.

There are three essential lessons that Jeff's life and death have taught me that I want to share with you:

- Each soul is important to God.
- Each soul is somebody's child, loved, dreamed for, and a promising possibility.
- Each soul is due the loving care of the local church.

When my shame was greatest and my pain was most acute, I decided to withdraw from our local church. Jeff came into my room that Sunday morning and challenged me. I will always remember his words: "Mama, I'm going to church to meet God!" Since God is only embodied in us, if Jeff had encountered you that morning, would he have met "God"?

My Rose

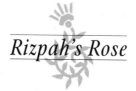

C h a p t e r 1

Rizpah's Rose

*D*i d you ever try to grasp something that was not really there? Have you ever tried to explain what you simply did not understand? Ever been in a fog, confused, frightened, and unsure of where you are or where you're headed? How do you feel when you are awakened from a sound sleep by a loud noise—in the dark, no lights and no clues as to what's there, frightened, scared, and fearful of the possibilities? Well, combine these puzzling instances, add the complexity of a mother's love, her child's illness, relations with others, and maternal care, and you have my story in a nutshell.

My story is one that is ages old and yet astonishingly fresh. With every telling the pain is original. For I am the mother of a son who was homosexual and died of the dread disease of AIDS. My tale is repeated daily, with only the names changed to protect outsiders from our painful realities. I think I always knew that Jeff was homosexual, but we never talked about it, for he was simply my child. Every homosexual is some mother's child. Invested in this blood relationship are hopes, dreams, plans, and much love. Homosexuals are not objects or things, but flesh-and-blood people with family ties.

Jeff was always sensitive, thoughtful, and excited about beautiful things. He had an artistic nature and was extra caring. His gentle and loving personality raised no red flags for me; he was completely my adoring and delightful son. He was a natural leader: opened the door for the nursery school bus driver, patrolled well as a patrol boy, led the way as the proud drum major for the high school band, founded a young people's choir while in college, took over office duties during his three years of military service, earned his master's degree, and formed a chapter of Omega Psi Phi, which is still going strong.

We never talked about Jeff being homosexual; he tried to hide this fact from me as long as possible. The last week of his life, he asked for his briefcase from home, then gave anything that might evidence his past into the hands of his niece and asked her to destroy it. He didn't want to hurt me. He tried so hard to protect me, while I was trying just as desperately to take his pain away. Jeff would give you the shirt off his back. And if he didn't have a shirt, he would take mine and give it to you! He tried so hard to be accepted, often resorting to "buying" the love he needed.

I can remember that Jeff came home on a trip with his college choir in 1983. He was not looking well to me. He had lost a lot of weight but said that he felt all right. I knew in my heart that something was wrong. When he returned to school he ended up in the hospital with hepatitis B for ten days. Jeff was probably positive for HIV (Human Immunodeficiency Virus) then. But I had never heard of HIV or AIDS and didn't have a clue how ill he was. The next thing I knew, Jeff called crying to tell me that he had been expelled from both the choir and the college band. He didn't give me a reason and I didn't ask. We both hid from further truth.

He was heartbroken over his expulsion from the activities he loved so well. We cried together over his pain, but we did not talk. When I went to North Carolina for his graduation, I started putting some of the very obvious pieces together as he introduced me to his friends. Shame was born within me. How I loved my son. And how I wanted him to be "normal" and just like everyone else. How could this have happened to my child? What went wrong? What had I done or neglected to do? All of the age-old questions reared their heads as I sat in the audience, trying to appear an "ordinary" mom. Yet somehow I knew that our lives would never be the same.

The African American community has a secret and unspoken fear about homosexuality. The names used for people who are "different" are vicious and ugly. Just as the majority culture has labeled and used negative stereotypes to define dissimilar cultural groups, so has my ethnic community taken this oppressive stance in our homophobic fears. I belong to the group. My thoughts and beliefs have been formed by them. I didn't know anything different. I had not sought additional information about the homosexual lifestyle, for in my family we were "normal, everyday people." As my reality became more distinctly clear, bad and sad feelings emerged, for I realized that my son was one of "them."

Jeff was the kindest and most loving person. He loved people, especially children. Following school Jeff entered the army. When he was discharged, he returned home to work with youngsters in a social service agency. He wanted to make a difference in their lives. But shortly after he started working, one of his cousins started a vicious lie that Jeff was molesting boys and he lost his job. The homophobic fears were at work even in our family. The son that I now had was not the son that I thought I had known.

One of my friends helped Jeff to get a new position with the city of Chicago. He hated working in personnel, but was soon promoted to supervisor in the youth division at the police department. Look at how God works! Our faith was strong and so was our denial! For we valiantly suppressed any further conversation about his homosexuality.

Jeff joined a major church in the city and became active in the sanctuary choir and the men's chorus. He was responsible for all of the music for the choirs and never missed a rehearsal. Whenever he became involved in something, I was included. So we both were faithful to the church and its many ministries. I needed some assurance that we were loved and accepted. I wanted to hear that Jeff was included in God's plan of salvation and redemption. I wanted some answers for my haunting questions about homosexuality. I wanted to feel understood, cared for, and sanctioned as a good mother, a good person, and a good Christian. But there was never any discussion of my particular situation. Not a word of hope was spoken to me or to Jeff. I felt so alone.

The story of Rizpah is recorded in the Scriptures. Second Samuel 21:1–14 details how this mother watched her only son be killed because of King Saul's sins years before the boy's birth. This mother loved her son and could not save his life. The verdict was pronounced and the death sentence carried out. Her child and six other young men were hanged from public gallows atop a high hill. The six corpses were left to decay as a sign of God's punishment for old sins. The Scriptures do not detail what happened to the other mothers. It only says that for a period of five months Rizpah stayed on the hill and protected the decaying bones of her son and the others.

Tennyson has written a poem titled "Rizpah." He puts these lines in her mouth: "Flesh of my flesh was gone, but bone of my bone was left—I stole them all . . . and you, will you call it a theft?" An artist, who only signed the name Turner, has painted a picture titled *Suffering* portraying Rizpah in ragged clothes, swinging an old tattered cloth with one hand as she fights off a buzzard and holding a torch in the other to keep a wild animal away from the decaying bones. I don't need the poem or the portrait. I know firsthand her pain of struggling to save what's left of her child. I understand completely her commitment to stay with him as long as possible. And I know how alone she was.

There is no record of a support group for her. No mention is made of other family members being considerate of her plight. Funny, but the community of faith is not referred to in her story. Like Rizpah, I was determined to be present for my child. Her love for the bones of her son speaks about the depth of her ties to the child she brought into the world. She was a mother and he was her rose. She was not standing alone, she was standing with her son. Like her, my family did not understand or appreciate my stance toward helping Jeff. And, like this biblical sister, the church had no solace for us.

Reflections

1. What is homophobia?
2. What is your theological position about homosexuality?
3. Are there known homosexuals in your family?
4. Are they loved and accepted by your family?
5. Are there known homosexuals in your church family?
6. Are they loved and accepted by your congregation?
7. Do you know of any support group for the families of homosexuals?
8. Do you feel they have a need for support and care? Why or why not?
9. Were you familiar with the suffering of Rizpah?
10. Do you know other mothers who have suffered with a dying child?

Chapter 2

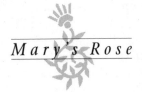

Mary's Rose

In early 1988 Jeff asked if one of his friends from Georgia could come to live with us until he and the friend got enough money for an apartment. With my husband having died two years before, the financial strain would have been too much. This was one time I said no. Jeff got so angry with me that he took his whole paycheck and sent it to his friend for a ticket to Chicago and arranged for him to live with other acquaintances. Furniture for their dream apartment was stored in my basement until they found the right place. The rent was astronomical. His friend didn't have a job and Jeff really could not afford it. So I ended up trying to take care of two households. I helped him buy a car, for his place was far away from me. We both struggled from payday to payday, but I didn't care. I knew that he would not be physically present for too many years.

We finally sat down and had a talk about AIDS. I begged him to be careful. He told me he could take care of himself. It was probably already too late, for July 11, 1989, Jeff called me at work and told me the doctor had diagnosed him as HIV-positive. God, how we cried on the phone. I wanted to go home, but the tears would not stop. Before I could leave, Jeff showed up in my office. He looked like a helpless child. With every fiber of my being I could hear him screaming, "Mama, help me!" My baby had just turned thirty the month before. What could I do?

We left the office and went to my home where we sat on the side of my bed and cried. He said that he was sorry he had hurt me. I was sorry that he was hurting too. He talked about how afraid he was. I was scared to death. He asked me to promise that I would not tell his siblings or anyone else about his diagnosis. I promised. I knew that I needed to talk with someone. I wanted to share my pain. But I promised to hold our secret and to swallow the pain. I could only talk to God, and believe me, I did that every single day.

Each morning when I arose, my affirmation was, "I can do everything through Him who gives me strength" (Philippians 4:13). Without holding on to my faith in God I would have disintegrated. My advice to Jeff was to eat right and take care of himself. I began to cook for him and even took food across the city to watch him eat. I tried to get him everything he wanted, for the smile on his face warmed by frightened heart.

The day he was diagnosed, I believe that Jeff set his appointment with death. But I never showed my emotions around him. As his mother, I was as alarmed as he was, but one of us had to be brave. I was the oldest. I was the wise one. I was going to get us through this somehow, some way. Did this seem like denial to me? Of course not! I was a mother who loved her child. I was a mother who must discover a way out for both of us. Isn't it true that "Mother knows best"?

I knew that this was a lie, but I began to educate myself on both homosexuality and AIDS. I ate books! It was startling to discover that a tiny organism called the Human Immunodeficiency Virus had been named in 1981. Most likely it has been around for much longer than that, for doctors on both the East and West Coasts became suspicious after having so many cases of strange pneumonias that would not clear up with normal antibiotics. It began to look like an epidemic. The similarity of each case, a male who admitted to having sex with another male, produced the misnomer "the gay plague." Each case reported the classic signs of a weakened natural defense system in the body. After much study it was revealed that HIV could be in the body for ten years before turning into AIDS. One of the common signs was rapid weight lost.

When Jeff started losing weight rapidly, I felt that every eye was on him. We stopped going to church services together, for I was busy watching the people watch my child. It got to the place where a member of the choir stopped me in the narthex one Sunday and asked, "Just what is wrong with Jeffery anyway?" I was so hurt I could not answer. I wanted to stop going to worship, but a dear friend and sister would pick me up every Sunday and refused to allow me the easy out of quitting. The stares were too much for me. The pain was unbearable. Jeff did not care what people thought, what they said, or how they looked at him. But my shame was overwhelming.

I felt as if AIDS had invaded only my family. Never were HIV or AIDS talked about from the pulpit or in any small group that I knew about. My shame drove me to isolation. The forced isolation became a fierce part of my hidden pain. Of course I have since discovered that shame and hiding are part of many lives in local congregations. My work with other families since Jeff's death has taught me that too many people come to church with their "smiley face" on to cover their hurts and fears. We live in a society where the media has told us to "never let them see you sweat!" So many families of ill loved ones come to God's house holding their secrets inside. How I longed for healing, support, and nurture. But I could not ask for help. And no one saw my pain. I continued to read, to gain knowledge, and to monitor Jeff.

By now I knew that AIDS was a sexually transmitted disease that had no cure and could be spread by both men and women, homosexual and heterosexual. The truth had emerged that AIDS was not just a disease limited to gays and drug users, but was affecting "straight" people also. In central Africa, the reports said that whole villages were being devastated by AIDS. The painful reality was that too many innocent babies were being infected even in their mothers' wombs. I don't know how all of this information had bypassed me before. But the more ill my baby became, the more I learned.

Jeff began to have mood swings. Sometimes I felt he even hated me. I would call to check on him and he would hang up. He told me that he hated to come around me because I was looking at him all the time. He would call me in the middle of the night, crying and talking about going away to get out of my life. There are no words to describe my feelings. I couldn't talk to anyone for I had made a promise. And even if the promise had not been made, I was too afraid to share this heavy burden. I was fearful people would reject Jeff. I was apprehensive that he would lose his job and then his apartment. I was alarmed about my own mounting anxieties.

By September Jeff had lost the vibrancy in his color. He was too sick to go to work at his full-time job. But with his friend not working and his concern over my financial struggle, Jeff took a part-time job at a fast-food restaurant as a manager. The staff at the restaurant were not kind. They treated him badly and someone broke out all the windows in his car. They were afraid and wanted him gone, but he remained there for six months until his health began to deteriorate rapidly.

In April of 1990 Jeff came to my home and showed me what he believed to be a boil on his inner thigh. It turned out to be a cyst on the lymph node that increased in size. Jeff was hospitalized with a form of cancer called lymphoma. His face started breaking out and there were big purple lesions on his chest. He went to a dermatologist, but the medicine made it worse. He tried to hide the skin problems by growing a beard. There were times when I went to pick him up from work and didn't recognize my own child. I felt like I was drowning and there was nobody around to help.

Mother's Day came and my daughter came home from California to surprise me. She brought my great-grandson and I was so uplifted and excited. The family planned a big dinner for me, but Jeff would not attend. How my feelings were hurt. But the family still did not know! The secret was yet being kept. I wanted to scream. I needed their support. But I had made Jeff a promise. Yet life cares nothing about our promises. And during this same time frame my aged father came to live with me, one daughter was in the process of foreclosure on her home, my other daughter was scheduled for surgery, and my granddaughter had gotten herself into serious trouble. I was so tired, so afraid and overwhelmed that I seriously considered suicide.

Jeff was tiring easily and had to rest after exerting any amount of energy. He tried to maintain his church life, took off driving to Ohio to a former pastor's installation, and went to Memphis with the choir. The summer was fairly quiet. He was taking his medicine and seemed to be looking better. He went to the emergency room because of breathing difficulties, but recovered and was released. I was hopeful. I wanted a miracle. I wanted him well.

In October he got sick in church one Sunday and had to leave. He got progressively worse. I took him to the doctors and they gave him more medicine. Wednesday, November 7, 1990, Jeff was diagnosed with full-blown AIDS. My world fell apart. I couldn't comprehend my child's impending death. I was angry with God. "Why, Lord? Jeff is so young. Why not me? I'm sixty-three. My baby is only thirty-three! Take me and please let him live."

I wonder if Mary tried to play "Let's Make a Deal" with God as she stood at the foot of the cross. Her child was only thirty-three. She had consented to bring him into the world. She had risked being stoned to death. Joseph had decided to divorce her privately. She had been homeless, a refugee, and a foreigner in order to keep Jesus alive. How did she feel standing there, watching her son die a slow and awful death?

All of the power of nature had reversed itself in order to make the Creator helpless and dependent upon her and Joseph. She had carried the Ancient of Days in her womb and nursed the Ruler of the Universe at her breast. It was her duty to teach him how to walk and talk. It was at her knees that he learned the faith of his ancestors. She had lulled him to sleep and watched over him as he grew. She had kissed the little hurts and made them better. And she had fixed his food and made a home for his earthly family. She was his mother. He was her son. Whatever happened to him also happened to her.

They had condemned him to death. They had mocked him at a false trial. They had flogged him and made him carry his own cross up the rugged hill. They had pounded nails into his hands and into his feet. She had heard his flesh tear. She had heard him cry out. She had watched him suffer. And she stood there at the foot of the cross. She couldn't kiss the "boo-boos" and make them better. She couldn't stroke the brow where the crown of thorns lay piercing his skin. She couldn't stop the pain or the agony. But she would be there for him to see her. She would stand with him as long as he was on this side of eternity. She would not faint or falter. In spite of the pain in her heart, she remained there for him to see. Mary's resolve to be present through it all was one I identified with easily. She became my model. She became my example. She became my ideal.

Jesus' friends had left him, with the exception of one. Those he had healed and fed and raised from the dead were absent from the crowd. But his mother was a fixture at the foot of his torture stake. She was his mother. He was her rose. I would not take the coward's way out and commit suicide. I could not leave Jeff to face this misery alone. Since he had to undergo this ordeal, he could depend upon me.

Reflections

1. Based on what you've read so far, was this mother codependent?

2. What would you have done in this situation?

3. What has another mother you know done in a similar situation?

4. What does your church provide for the family of HIV/AIDS patients?

5. What could your church provide?

6. What do you think about the mother's promise to keep Jeff's secret?

7. What can the church do to make it safe to share secrets of this nature?

8. Are you involved in keeping family secrets?

9. Did you ever try to imagine what Mary felt like on that Good Friday?

10. Have you ever walked with a loved one through the "valley of the shadow of death"?

R u t h 's   R o s e

*T*he Centers for Disease Control and Prevention, located in Atlanta, reported that in 1995 the number of AIDS cases among black children age twelve and under doubled. The number of black women infected through heterosexual contact or intravenous drug use increased during the same period. At the end of 1995, the reporting year, African Americans, who account for only 12.5 percent of the total population, made up 33 percent of the total HIV-infected population. The African American community now has the highest percentage, in all categories, of those who are contracting and dying from AIDS.

Yet my community and my church were virtually silent on the issue. The facts that I had came from books and the media. Even though I kept a daily journey, I could not write the word "AIDS" in it. I simply called it "bad news." I was afraid of the word. There was little information available about African American male homosexuals. With all of the stereotypical myths about black male sexual prowess, homosexuality seemed a contradiction. Sexuality of any type was not discussed openly, so the issue of homosexuality and a spreading vicious disease was a closed topic.

My lack of information and my pledge to secrecy fed my denial of Jeff's terminal condition. I really did not believe that God would take Jeff away from me. I knew within my heart of hearts that my son would have a miraculous healing. However, Jeff knew better.

When the virus in his body turned into full-blown AIDS, Jeff knew that he needed the most popular medicine, Zidovudine (commonly called AZT), which is the major drug used to slow the progress of HIV in the body. He was afraid to get it on his health insurance for fear of discovery and termination. In an already tight financial crunch, we began to pay about four hundred dollars a month for prescriptions.

Jeff discovered that as he took the meds, he tired more easily. But he continued to do the things he had always done. He played volleyball on Saturdays, attended fraternity meetings, went out with friends on weekends, didn't come in till late, got up early for church, and generally wasn't getting proper rest. He cut his meds in half to conserve his energy and would not stop the dangerous treadmill pace. I was worried crazy and plagued with financial woes. Most of my money went into things for Jeff.

We made it till the end of 1990 and went to church for Watch Night Service. Jeff was so ill that it was difficult for him to attend. That night my pastor preached a sermon titled "Learning to Embrace Real Change." He told us that there were three parts to change. The first is fear. The second is fact. He instructed us to concentrate on the condition and not on our position. Finally, he addressed the issue of our faith. I listened closely, straining to embody every word. I wrote down the key points. He was talking directly to me and to Jeff.

After worship, Jeff was so weak that we went immediately home. I had to help him undress. I began to acknowledge his "change." I went into my room and cried into the new year. With faith, I continued by the grace of God, doing all of my many tasks. Although my mind, body, spirit, and soul were in a constant whirl with the required activities, I had to go on. Even when I knew that my own mental and physical health were not receiving proper attention, I was able to continue giving care to others.

As we entered another year, it became more and more of a struggle for me to walk into my local church. When we would walk into church together, I could "feel" the whispers. I thought about resigning from all of my positions. "Who needs this aggravation?" I asked myself. And I told Jeff how I felt. He replied that no one was going to stop him from going to church but God. He told me that he needed me to go with him. I prayed for the strength to continue.

The many hats I wore continued to increase as Jeff found it too tiring to drive. So I would pick him up and deliver him wherever he had to go. Trips to the hospital were becoming more frequent as a new problem arose every day. He hadn't worked a full week in months. Office gossip began. When he told me about this, I was angry. Where could my child be accepted? I was already worried about the stares at church, and now even outsiders were beginning to shun him. I just wanted to scream.

As the illness became more severe, I became more agitated with Jeff's live-in friend. He had never found a job. He didn't seem to care about Jeff's failing health. And he began to take advantage of Jeff's car as if he owned it. Along with all of the other problems in our lives, I greatly resented him. He was not even being a good friend. And if there was ever a time, this was the period when my child needed a true friend.

Ruth taught me much about the covenant of friendship. Basically she said, "Where you go, I will go; and where you stay, I will stay. Your people will be my people, and your God my God" (Ruth 1:16). She vows before God to be faithful, dependable, and completely linked to another's life. She makes a pact between herself and the woman who has become her mother-in-law, Naomi.

Naomi's husband and two sons died in a foreign land, leaving her with two daughters-in-law to be responsible for as head of the house. When a famine comes along, with no male providers, these women are vulnerable and uncertain. Naomi decides to return to her homeland. At the crossroads, she tries to persuade the two women to return to their parents' homes. I know she was tired of mothering and nurturing. I know she had come to the end of her wits trying to feed three mouths and discover new ways to stretch what was not there. Orpah followed her admonition and stayed at the crossroads. Ruth, however, made a promise to bind her life to Naomi's and to follow her destiny.

The contract that Ruth made was based on their friendship and not their blood kinship. Friendship caused Ruth to willingly become a foreigner in a strange land. Friendship caused a younger woman to become mother to an older woman. Friendship caused a woman to give up her culture and her ethnic identity. Friendship is about loyalty, devotion, and allegiance. Friendship is a decision. And friendship is challenged in times of personal crisis.

I am persuaded that the stories in the Bible are there to show us how God acts in our lives. Ruth modeled God in remaining close to Naomi. Ruth stood alongside a woman who was in turmoil, dealing with a catastrophe in her life. Naomi felt that God had abandoned her in taking away her husband and sons. A woman was considered nothing if she had no man in her life. So Naomi felt helpless and thought victim's thoughts. "Don't call me Naomi. . . . Call me Mara, for the Almighty has made my life very bitter." Yet in risking to return home alone, God gave her Ruth with a covenant of friendship.

Jeffery was facing the biggest challenge of his life. His attitude said that God was with him. If his so-called companion didn't know how to be a friend, I did.

Reflections

1. In times of personal crisis, who is there for you?

2. Who are the people in your life who are dependable and loyal?

3. Who are the church friends who have proven their vows of fellowship?

4. What makes people friends?

5. Do we really need people as friends when we have God in our lives?

6. Can a parent be a true friend?

7. Is there a difference between society's and the church's expectation of friends?

8. How do you feel about having friends who are gay and lesbian?

9. How do you feel about Ruth's covenant of friendship?

10. Can a person with AIDS count on your friendship?

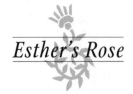

Esther's Rose

*F*ebruary of 1991 found me reading Isaiah 43:2 as my daily affirmation. It promised, "When you pass through the waters, I will be with you; and when you pass through the rivers, they will not sweep over you. When you walk through the fire, you will not be burned, the flames will not set you ablaze." My prayer life increased as I challenged God: "Where are you? Are you going to keep this promise? Were you talking to me? I'm drowning in rivers of difficulty!"

One night after prayer I had the strangest dream. I dreamed I was driving home and as I came close to my house, it seemed as though my eyesight was dimming and I just could not see. I bypassed my home. As soon as I realized what had occurred, there were blue flashing police lights behind me. I stopped and turned off the ignition. The officer tapped on the window, so I started the car in order to roll down the window. I never saw the officer's face, only from his waistline down. Yet this public servant knew all about me, where I lived and worked, about my family and church, even that I was a deacon. The question was asked of me, "Why did you pass by your house?" I responded that I could not see it. The radio was on and I was instructed to call the radio station. I don't know where a phone came from, but as I called, the officer disappeared. I began to drive again, and it seemed that every direction ended at a dead-end street. I was completely lost. I decided to get out of the car and walk, and I found myself in the middle of a desert. There were no houses or people, just the wilderness and me. I started crawling through miles of dirt and crawled for what seemed like hours. I began to pray out loud for God's help. A house appeared on the top of a hill. As I began to crawl up the hill, I met a group of women jogging. One told me that she was a helicopter pilot and that she would take me home. I awoke thanking and praising God for helping me while I was in the wilderness.

My resolve to walk with Jeff to the very conclusion of this ordeal was strengthened. Knowing that what lay ahead was going to be much worse than what we had already experienced, I was determined not to let my child see me falter in my faith. My help was coming from somewhere. I was lost and could not see my way. But the God of heaven and earth was going to get me through this wilderness experience. I began to understand Proverbs 3:5: "Trust in the Lord with all your heart; and lean not on your own understanding." The journey that I was on was not based on knowledge and facts; it was based on faith in God.

The day after my dream, the doctor told Jeff that his T-cell count was increasing. After being off work for a week, he was able to return. That Thursday, Jeff met me at work for a ride to choir rehearsal. He told me that he was through taking medicine, even though he knew that without it he would die. He began to encourage me to talk about his impending death, funeral arrangements, and what he wanted me to have from his apartment. When I got to my bedroom and closed the door, I fell down on my knees. "Lord, are you really going to put me through this? I can't bear it!"

Jeff had good days and bad ones. He would call me all night long. His whole personality was changing. He was angry with the world, everything in it, and with me. He fought constantly with his friend and got so angry that I thought he would kill himself with either a massive stroke or heart attack.

That summer Jeff applied for a flight attendant's position, which he'd always wanted. He passed the preliminary test and was asked to travel out of town for an interview. I told him that this was an impossibility. He not only went for the first interview, but went again for a second one. How great is our God! Then they set a date for a physical. I asked God to work it out, because we knew he couldn't pass the examination.

Jeff began to worry about going over the specified weight limits. He quit eating food completely and drank a liquid diet three times a day. I begged and pleaded with him to eat. I tried to talk sense into him about how he was further stressing his body. He would not listen. Of course the end result was that he got so weak he couldn't go to take the physical. He cried. I cried. I could see my child dying right before my very eyes.

His health was deteriorating so rapidly that he was only working a couple of days a week. I don't know how he did it. I begged him to take a leave of absence and get some rest. He would not give up trying to work in order to prevent me further financial strain. He would not give up going to church or to choir rehearsals. Even though he was too weak to sing, he would go and listen to the others rehearse.

We went to his sister's house for Thanksgiving dinner. He didn't eat because he couldn't. He lay on the couch the entire day. But he wanted to be there. It was to be his last one with us. Every time we were alone, Jeff wanted to talk about his death. I didn't listen. I told him that I didn't want to talk about it. He informed me that he was no longer afraid, and he encouraged me to face reality for his sake.

As I kept praying, wishing, and hoping, Jeff kept making his funeral arrangements without my knowledge. Later I discovered that he had called everyone he wanted to be involved in his funeral and gave them specific instructions.

As the Christmas holidays approached, Jeff told me he wanted a black tree with green and red decorations as a gift. He told me where to find it, but he didn't know how much it cost. I found the tree and called to tell him that with decorations the cost was three hundred dollars. He told me to forget it for the cost was too great. I got it anyway and I'm glad that I did. Three weeks before Christmas I surprised him with it. He cried when I took him to pick it up. He put it up that night. He adored that beautiful tree. Then he came to put up a tree at my house. It would be the last time I would have a Christmas tree. It took him so long—he stopped often to rest. He didn't want my help; he wanted to do it himself. He knew that this was the last time he would perform this task of love.

He had been too ill to shop, but one of his friends had taken him to the mall and then brought him to my house, where we had to help him to bed. He marched in with the choir during worship on Christmas morning. As he came past me, on the front row, he put a wrapped gift in my lap. I didn't open it. When we came home from church, he told me that he'd wanted me to have the gift in church for it was a computerized King James Version of the Bible. It was his last Christmas gift to me.

The last time that Jeff and I prayed together in worship was at the New Year's Eve service, 1991. I don't remember the sermon my pastor preached; it was one of the few times I did not write it down. What stands out in my mind about that night is that we prayed in the New Year together, right in front of the altar, next to the podium. There was Jeff, his sister, his niece and nephew, and me. Next to us was my pastor and his family. Pastor's baby daughter kept hugging Jeff. I said, "Thank you, Lord." Here was a little child, and she wasn't afraid to touch him. It brought a big smile to my baby's face. "God, how I give you praise."

The next day, in the midst of all the activities, I did remember the title of the Reverend's sermon. It was "Words That Make a Difference." Although I didn't remember any of the words "that make a difference," I recalled some other significant words: "When you go through rivers of difficulty, you will not drown."

Esther faced tremendous difficulties. The odds against her and her people were overwhelming. Yet she had an inner resolve that saved all of their lives. She had a few things to teach me. Like me, Esther was keeping a secret. No one knew that she was a Jew. Her cousin Mordecai had ordered her not to reveal her ethnic identity (Esther 2:20). She had been made queen by King Ahasuerus of Persia because of her beauty.

One of the king's princes, Haman, hated Jews in general and hated Mordecai in particular. He conspired to have the king decree the death of every Jew. The king signed the decree and the death order became official. Letters were drawn up in the name of the king and sent to every province "with the order to destroy, kill, and annihilate all the Jews, young and old, women and little children . . . and to plunder their goods" (Esther 3:12–13).

When the word began to circulate, the people of Persia were confused and the Jewish communities went into "great mourning . . . with fasting and weeping and wailing. Many of them lay in sackcloth and ashes" (4:3). While death was being planned, the queen sat safely in the palace. But the word of death travels fast, and her ladies in waiting told her that Mordecai was in front of the palace in great distress. When she discovered the reason for his grief and sent him clothes, he sent back a message to her: "Do not think that in the king's palace you will escape any more than all the other Jews. For if you keep silence at such a time as this, relief and deliverance will rise for the Jews from another quarter, but you and your father's family will perish. Who knows but that you have come to royal position for such a time as this" (4:13–14).

Talk about a time of wrestling with a decision. Talk about a period of struggling with choices. Talk about a whirl of thoughts passing through her mind as she grappled with the issues before her. But words make a difference. "Who knows but that you have come to royal position for such a time as this." Esther resolved to do what she could to save her loved ones. She put her fate in God's hands as she called for the Jews and her ladies in waiting to fast with her for discernment of a strategy. She recognized that she was in a position of great difficulty. But she was fortified with faith that she would not drown.

A crisis always calls forth choices from us. The Chinese symbols for crisis and for opportunity are one and the same. Esther saw the crisis as an opportunity to rely on God's intervention. Finally her words made a difference. For she moved forth saying, "I will go to the king . . . and if I perish, I perish" (4:16). Under extremely difficult circumstances Esther's resolve saved lives. Just as Mordecai's words struck a responsive cord in Esther's heart, my pastor's sermon hit home in mine.

Reflections

1. Can you recall a time when you felt lost and in a desert place?
2. How did God reach you with comfort?
3. Is there significance for daily life in dreams?
4. What biblical affirmations can be prayed by those with AIDS?

5. What biblical affirmations can be prayed by the loved ones of those with AIDS?

6. What difficult period in your life can you use to give hope to those facing death?

7. Why have you "come to royal position for such a time as this"? What role is God requiring of you in the position you're in now?

8. As you analyze the dream, who was the officer, who were the joggers, and why was she lost in wilderness/desert?

9. If you had known of this mother-son journey, what help would you have offered during this crisis period?

10. What are the words that have made a difference in your life?

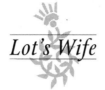

Lot's Wife

The very first Sunday in January, Jeff called and told me that he had blood in his urine. He told me that he was scared for the first time in many weeks. I was getting ready for church and didn't know what to do. He called to tell me to go on to church, for he would meet me there. He called me later from his car phone and asked me to turn the radio on. As I found the station, the announcer said that Jeffery Bell had requested a song for his mother. "I feel like going on! I feel like going on! Though trials come on every hand, I feel like going on!" I didn't know if I could go on. I surely didn't want to endure this trial. But Jeff needed me by his side. This was his affirmation. So I drove to church in tears.

That Monday the hospital called and said they had scheduled a biopsy due to the swelling in his upper thigh. Jeff was having constant stomach pains and could not walk straight. He was bent over like an old man. The doctor told him he was suffering the consequences of not taking his medicine. He went to his apartment and called me every hour, all night long, telling me how sick he was. He was begging for my help.

All night long I had to listen to the pleas of my child and there was nothing I could do but pray. I knew that God was his only help, but I wanted to offer more than prayers. I needed to have something that could make him feel better, take the pains away, stop his misery. My helplessness tore me up. My heart felt as though it would literally break in two. My nerves were taut, my spirit low, and my hopes almost dissipated as I listened to the agonizing appeals that I could not answer.

The last time he called me that night, he told me that he couldn't take it anymore and was going to commit suicide. What could I say? He knew he was dying. The sheer fright of living with AIDS was enough to kill him or anybody else. Have you ever thought how it feels to live with a time bomb within your system? Whenever he showered, he saw the lesions that are the telltale signs of Kaposi's sarcoma, the form of skin cancer associated with AIDS. Every time he coughed, caught a cold or a fever, it became a possibility of impending disaster. Being tired all of the time and having to give up the activities that he loved was a living death to my active son. I told him that I was praying and asked him to pray too.

Every day after that felt like a precious gift from God. The next weekend Jeff spent with me so that he could more easily attend church that Sunday. I couldn't go. I had reached my limits. Bed was the best worship I could receive. That night Jeff called and said he was sick and coming to pick me up to go to the hospital. I got up, dressed, and waited. When he did not show up, I panicked. "What if he's had an accident?" I went absolutely mad.

At 8:30 P.M. his sister called me from California. Jeff had gone to the hospital, checked himself in, and called her to ask her to call me. He had not told her which hospital! I couldn't begin to figure out where he might be, north side or south side of town. Finally he called me, but would not tell me where he was. He was concerned that I was already too tired. He promised to call when he was released the next day.

It was 1:30 A.M. when he called to say the doctor had told him that nothing more could be done except taking more pain pills. At 2:30 A.M. he called again, despondent. He said some horrible, hurtful things to me because I wouldn't help him commit suicide. I told him that I loved him too much to even think of assisting him. There was no reasoning with him. But if the doctors had told me to live with constant pain and wait for death, how would I have felt? I had no clue. And the fact that some brain studies of AIDS victims showed significant damage due to destruction of brain cells by the virus was no small thing. So I cried and prayed. And I prayed and cried. Later, before dawn, he called to tell me that the pain had subsided. Thanks be unto God!

On Wednesday we went to the outpatient clinic for the biopsy. One of the associates from our church came to be with Jeff, and the nurse was also one of our church members. God was trying to reach me with support, but I couldn't feel it. I was numb and mindless. After a while you become overwhelmed with the constant grief and stress of trying to cope with a situation that will not get better. The secrecy, the guilt, the shame, and the isolation were eating away at my insides. I felt like I was going to explode.

We were at the hospital from 10:30 A.M. to 3:30 P.M. When we left, the car was covered with ice, the doors frozen. I was concerned about Jeff being out in that weather after surgery, so I told him to stay inside while I got help. We had to stop and get a prescription filled for the pain pills. Since Jeff had to remain inside for at least twenty-four hours, he went home with me. Thank God a friend stopped by, in zero weather, to bring us food. I was totally exhausted.

When I got Jeff to bed, my father begin rehearsing a too familiar tune: "You had better spend some time with me, for I'll be checking out soon!" Will somebody tell me when this ends? "God, give me strength," I prayed. I went to work the next day feeling that Jeff would sleep because of the anesthesia. Instead of him calling me all day, my father did. He needed to know how to turn off the radio. Did I have anything for him to eat? (As though I did not cook and feed him every single day!) He called and told me he had fallen and couldn't get up. (Watching commercials too much?) I called my neighbor, bless her heart, who went to see about him. I couldn't figure out why Daddy was falling so often. I took him to the doctor who could find no explanation. Later I discovered the reason. It was a bottle of brandy hidden in his room! "Lord, I don't think I'm going to make it!"

Here I was taking care of the father who had been responsible for me and caring for the child I brought into the world. I was trying to envision a future for my son while holding on to some old resentments against my father. I was caught in the middle. At times I didn't know whether I was coming or going. Many times it felt like I was walking on Jell-O. My father wanted my attention and my son needed my strength. Who was there for me? Did anybody see my needs?

Jeff was asleep when I left for work that Friday and God knew he needed the rest. He seemed to have so much courage. I wished again that I could bear this pain for him. He called me later in the day to say that Daddy had fallen again. He had called my brother, who couldn't come. But when I got home Daddy had gotten into bed and was complaining that his side hurt. But he managed to get up for dinner.

That night I called my daughter in California. I had not heard from her recently. I felt that she was angry with me for doing so much for Daddy and Jeff. She had no idea how sick Jeff was and I couldn't tell her. I just prayed that she would call Jeff and perhaps he would tell her. Of course she did not. I couldn't stop thinking about the relationship between my daughter in California and Jeff. I hoped that someday she would understand why I did what I could. It was so difficult for me to see my child ill and suffering. She would have had to be here, to live here, to walk in my shoes in order to understand. My world was going in circles. My energy level was almost nonexistent. But I was determined to go on.

It was Sunday morning and I was going to church. I guess I really looked down. I was. Everyone kept asking me what was wrong. I told all the polite lies and made it through worship. When I got home, Jeff was in his room crying. He came to my room with a handful of pills and told me that he was going to take them all. I told him that I could not stop him, it was his choice, but it would be without my help or my blessing. The power to speak to him with force and conviction came from someplace within that I cannot identify. There were no tears. There was no anger. There was simply a calm. He heard me, loud and clear, and returned to his room.

Jeff's friend had his car but no money to buy gas and phoned to tell Jeff that he needed to get some money. On my way out the door with some friends to dinner, I instructed Jeff to have him leave the car parked in front of my house. This money machine was empty! Daddy began to complain that the house was cold while the thermostat was up on eighty. He really wanted me to stay at home. But I needed some down time. I was tired, tired, tired. I prayed for strength to make it through the dinner.

When I arrived home, the police were parked in front of my house. I thought I would faint. My mind starting to race. Had Jeff committed suicide? What was happening? I was afraid to enter my own home. Inside I discovered that Jeff had called the police because his friend was determined to take his car. I asked the friend to leave, and he left on foot. The police left. By this time Daddy was complaining that his side was hurting from the many falls, and Jeff was down on his knees crying because his stomach was hurting.

I went to the drugstore for more pain pills, got Daddy to bed, had to go back to my office to pick up a package, and thought about running away. Running women are not new. Trying to get away from madness is not strange. The inability to handle the pressures have caused many stronger women than I to head off into the wild, blue yonder. I thought about Lot's poor, nameless wife and the way Renita Weems tells her story in *Just a Sister Away*. Weems says the woman "was not looking back, she was just looking around!"

I had looked around for so long, searching for some method, some strategy, some tactic that would bring me some mental, emotional, and spiritual release. I had thought of my mother. She had been abused by my father for so long. With the birth of her last child, she had sworn she would leave him when the child was eighteen. And, on that very day, she moved out of the state. But look how long she had suffered, endured, and held on to fading hopes and broken promises before she ran away to life.

I looked at my own courtship and marriage. It had started off so well. He seemed such a gentleman, courteous and decent. Was I fooled? I had married my father! For thirty-eight years I had survived a life of verbal abuse and emotional anguish. Ultimatums, demands, and dictates were the normal course of my every day. He was angry. He was vicious. He was hardhearted. Never any kind words or nice deeds. No presents or tokens of affection. Just a mean spirit and ugly attitude. Then he got sick and died. That had been my only escape.

I looked to my church, where I was faithful, consistent, and hardworking. I went to church looking for a caring and nurturing community. We belonged to a large congregation, but we were known by the small inner groups with which we served. The people came Sunday after Sunday to sing, praise, and shout. The music was lively, the crowd was stimulated, and the worship was enjoyed. But people kept their eyes closed to our constant pain. People reached out to embrace us, but did not touch our inner selves. People asked how we felt, but did not hear our true response. They sang of working in the realm of God but hurried past so as not to get actively involved. They prayed for hope and healing but did not want to be the instrument God would use. They read and heard the Scriptures but never received the word of Jesus that would open up their hearts and cause them to pour out the love that had been flooded into them. My child was fading right before their eyes. They refused to see. My heart was broken, my countenance had changed, and I was running wildly, looking for genuine Christian compassion. The church people had on blinders and were busy telling gentle, polite lies as they ignored our plight. Now I was between a father I had always resented and a son that I did not know, but had always loved. They both needed me. I was always available to them. The question was, who would care for me?

I understood Lot's wife and her need to look around. Most likely she was asking herself where she was. She had no name that we have ever heard. She most likely felt that she had no "self," no personhood, no identity outside her man and her family. Every woman has a need to stop and look around, for it's possible to lose yourself. Or maybe the pillar of salt came from stopping along the way to cry and grieve for the woman she could have been.

Reflections

1. Who cares for caregivers in your community?
2. Find out what you can about "respite sites" in your area.
3. When the doctors say "there is nothing more we can do," how can the church continue to minister?
4. What is your church's teaching on suicide?
5. How do you feel about assisted suicide?
6. What situation has rendered you both "numb and mindless"?
7. Is there less shame and guilt associated with cancer than with AIDS?

8. Do people openly talk about cancer and its effects in your community?

9. If "it takes a village to raise a child," how many does it take to care for an aging parent?

10. What can the church offer to caregivers who just need to "look around"?

Chapter 6

My Wilting Rose

*M*onday, January 20, 1992, my oldest son turned forty-two. I called him in California to wish him a happy birthday. We made it through the day with few episodes. Jeff's friend came by at midnight and needed a ride to the apartment. Jeff was too weak to stand up and I wasn't going anywhere.

Wednesday of that week we got the results of the biopsy. Jeff had cancer too. We cried all day long. He did tell his sister who lives here in the city, and she joined us in tears. Our pastor called long-distance to see how Jeff was getting along. My deacons group called from their meeting at the church. People were reaching out. Cancer was a safe word to talk about. It was acceptable. Regardless, I needed the support. I felt that I had nothing left within.

This news could be shared with my daughter in California. She called Jeff, apologized for her behavior, and they talked a long time. Jeff went back to work. I wasn't getting enough sleep, for I knew the truth and how complicated Jeff's care was going to be. Yet I had to go to work. My friend Doris picked me up and helped me prepare for my board meeting. I worked and cried all day. Honestly, I don't know how I got through it.

Jeff came home with me after work so he could go to rehearsal. One of his friends picked him up. It was snowing, he was tired, but he went to choir practice. Later someone told me that Jeff testified that night and asked folks to pray for me. What kind of man is that? A caring and compassionate son. He spent the night at my house.

That Friday morning I fixed breakfast and dinner for Daddy before going to work. Jeff was getting dressed and I stopped to watch him. His clothes were so big on him. I had just bought them. My child had been a big, strapping, good-looking man. He had broad shoulders and wore beautifully tailored clothes. When I saw what this disease had done to him, my heart hurt and my tears began to flow. Still I gave God the glory for what little strength he had left. I wondered how he was holding on.

Doris was such a true friend, in every sense of the word. She never asked probing questions, but made it her business to look out for me however she could. She picked me up for work and had no idea of what a blessing it was not to drive. On this particular day, she left the parking ticket in the car as usual. When we got ready to go home that night, we could not find the ticket. She had put it in the ashtray, as was her custom, but it had disappeared. We had to explain to the cashier about the ticket, for there was a twenty dollar charge for a lost ticket. The cashier didn't charge us. We got the best laugh about the disappearing ticket. Proverbs says that a merry heart can do you as good as medicine. I needed that laugh. I couldn't remember laughing in months. The laughter reminded me that God was still at work.

I awoke the next morning crying. I couldn't keep the tears out of my eyes. It had snowed the night before, and after eating breakfast, Jeff decided he would go outside and shovel the snow for me. I cried some more. He wanted to do it, but we both knew he didn't have the strength. Doris went shopping for our weekend needs, and my daughter came over with her son to shovel the walkways. Then she challenged me to come outside for a snowball fight. The gift of laughter returned.

That Sunday morning I decided that church and I would part company. I was tired of the looks and whispers. Jeff came into my room to see if I was dressed for worship. I told him that I couldn't take it anymore. He told me something that I will never forget. He said, "Mama, I'm going to church to meet God. And I don't care what the people say or do! I'm going!" I got up and went with him. He decided to stay for both services, but I came home to get some sleep. His sister brought him home and prepared dinner for all of us.

Jeff's eyes were starting to turn as red as fire. Every day there seemed to be a different problem. At 11:40 P.M., Jeff came to tell me that since he had no clothes for work, he was going to his apartment. The weather was bad and I began to pray. He called to let me know that he made it home. I was up at 5:00 A.M. to balance my checkbook and pay the mounting bills. The house was a mess, but I had nothing in me to address its state. I called to tell Doris not to pick me up, for Jeff had a doctor's appointment. She said I sounded so tired that she would come anyway. When Jeff arrived, we left to get him to the doctor's office. They removed the stitches from the biopsy and he was in pain the rest of the day. I came down with a cold, the first I'd had in many years.

Monday we had a consultation with a cancer specialist. Jeff was scheduled for a CAT scan. He was getting weaker every passing day, his blood count stayed low, and his hands and feet remained as cold as ice. He drove me to work and went on to the clinic to see his medical doctor. Of all things, Doris's car quit on her and she had to have it towed to the dealership. Jeff went to pick her up, but her car was ready and he had to make the return trip alone. She trailed him home, but he kept getting sick. I kept in touch with him by car phone, but I was so scared. He kept calling to say that he couldn't make it. I was going crazy. All I could do was pray, pray, and pray. He made it home.

Wednesday, January 29, 1992, was my sixty-third birthday. I felt every year. I was sick. I was tired. I was physically exhausted. I got up and went to work. My coworkers had planned a luncheon for me, but I just had no party spirit. I asked them to postpone it for another time. Jeff had stayed home from work due to extreme fatigue. A dozen red roses and a dozen happy birthday balloons were delivered from him to my office. They didn't cheer me up. My heart became more grieved with sadness, for I knew that this was my last birthday he would be here to celebrate. Jeff had sent me roses for every one of my birthdays since he turned eighteen. How I cried. "Lord, I can't stand it. Have you deserted me too?"

The next morning I awoke at 5:00 A.M., hearing my name faintly called. It was Jeff and he was in terrible pain. I was at my wit's end. I had no more answers and could not pull up any reserve hope. I knew I was supposed to do something. Heaven knows that I'm his mother. An adage goes "life is like a tea bag, and your strength comes in hot water." My water couldn't get any hotter! I gave Jeff a bath, rubbed him down, fixed him a cup of tea, and gave him some pain pills. Then I left for work.

Work had become my salvation. Work was the only thing that would get my mind off all of the pressing problems. Work kept me from having to constantly watch Jeff and hear Daddy's growing list of complaints. Work forced me to have a clear head in order to be responsible for a three million dollar budget for my agency. The easiest thing in the world for me to do was go to work.

When I came home that evening, Daddy met me saying he had been waiting all day for me to fix him some food. The food was prepared, sitting in the refrigerator on a plate, waiting for him to microwave it for ninety seconds. I was so stressed that my body broke out in boils. (Ever hear of

Job?) I had a boil so big on my waistline that I could hardly wear any clothes. I realized that I needed to see a doctor. But I saw so many doctors with Jeff and Daddy that I'd had more than enough of them.

When Jeff came home later than evening he was in terrible pain. I told him that every pain he had, I had too. He took a bath, and would not listen as I tried to prevent him from taking a walk in zero weather. When he shut the door, I burst out in tears. They were tears of tiredness, frustration, and hopelessness. I had a sick son who was going crazy and taking me right along with him.

The only way to deal with this situation was to take both him and me to Jesus. There was a mother in Matthew 15 and Mark 7 whose love for an ill daughter drove her to find relief. I clearly understood this woman's need for restoration, healing, and hope. For a crisis in your home is hell. It demands your full and immediate attention. Work and church were important issues in my life and had their share of problems and distress. But this was the most overwhelming situation I had ever faced.

This nameless woman, who stands for me and all the other mothers who have lost their children to unnamed diseases, entered the life of Jesus at the point when the church people had driven him into hiding. While they were planning and plotting to take his life, this mother was looking for someone who could rescue her and her child from a pressing danger. In verse 25, Mark records: "A woman whose little daughter was possessed by an evil spirit came and fell at his feet." Mark informs us that Jesus and the disciples were hiding in a home attempting to avoid discovery. And into this clandestine gathering intruded this audacious, bold, and brash woman. She not only brought all of her years of baggage and pain, but she brought the illness of her child.

She was not a "church lady," not a converted believer,

and not even a Jew. But she had tried all the traditional cures and none of them had helped her child. Now her daughter's salvation was her first priority, for the hell in her house had forced her to seek additional assistance. It made her no difference that she was coming with all types of strikes against her, being both foreign and female. She simply knew that with her own set of personal issues, dynamics, and problems, she must have divine intervention of some sort.

There is no history of how long the daughter had been afflicted. But the progression of your child's illness always has you struggling to see some little sign of recovery. And the chief tool of the enemy of our soul is deep despair. When we become convinced that the situation we are in is hopeless, we want to give up on God and the church. We still go to worship, we sing the songs, we might say the creeds, but we really don't believe that God cares. When despair sets in we can become so focused on our personal limits that we forget that God has no limits. This foreign woman refused to believe that Jesus was restricted to providing miracles for the Jews. She wanted her own.

Matthew 15:22 records: "Lord, Son of David, have mercy on me." Her plea was mine. It's an impassioned supplication for aid. Then she cried out, "My daughter is suffering terribly." The petition has two distinct parts that are intertwined. Even though she recognized her own need for healing, she sought aid for her child. And verse 23 is a kick in her face, for it says, "Jesus did not answer a word."

Jesus was silent. Jesus was quiet. Jesus was hushed and still. The silence had to have been disturbing to her. I know that not receiving answers to my prayers confused me. The silence is distressing, perplexing, and remote. Often it's impossible to discern what's happening in the midst of heaven's silence. So I cried. The tears spoke volumes. The tears released all I was holding within. The tears washed my lamenting spirit. Like this mother, I grieved for my son and I grieved for myself. How glad I am that I was able to cry.

Years ago someone wrote the song "Big Girls Don't Cry!" Yet, as I think back over my journey with Jeff, tears were good companions. Tears helped me to relieve the inner stress and let go of what I could not control or change. There is a need for good grief. There is a place in our lives for appropriate anguish and sadness. In order to take good care of our emotional self, sometimes even "big girls" have to cry! I'm glad this biblical sister cried out for attention from Jesus. He met her needs. He also met mine.

When my wounded heart and broken spirit were not recognized by others, Jesus was paying close attention to my needs. Although I never got a loud, immediate, verbal response, like this sister, I learned how to wait on God. The hymn writer Adelaide Pollard says it best for us:

> Have thine own way, Lord!
> Have thine own way!
> Thou art the Potter; I am the clay.
> Mold me and make me after thy will,
> While I am *waiting,* yielded and still.

Love held me in the silence. God's Word instructed me in the silence. God's Holy Spirit energized me in the silence. And God's amazing grace kept me sane. On Friday, January 31, I stayed home from work, sick from the cold, the boils, and Jeff's misery. I received a card that day from my boss's wife. It let me know that God had people caring for me, praying for me, and taking me before the throne of God, even though they didn't know my inner pain. God spoke through her love.

I was elected to the board of deacons that night. Both Jeff and I were absent. Another sister had to stand up for me when they called my name. I was so angry with God. I didn't feel worthy of an office in the church. Yet it was on this night that Jeff thanked me for staying home with him that day. He said it made him feel good. I didn't know he felt that way. In the silence, God was speaking the language of love.

At the end of the story Jesus told the woman, "Daughter, your faith has made you whole." Her great faith moved Jesus to respond. Her majestic faith won the victory. Her notable faith teaches us how to hold steady in the face of every opposition. Her majestic faith inspires us to be relentless when it seems that there is no answer to our dilemma. At the time, I didn't feel as if I had "great faith." Now I know that I did.

Reflections

1. Has laughter ever been "good medicine" for you?
2. Has crying ever been therapeutic for you?
3. Have you had to watch a loved one "waste away" before your eyes?
4. What/who helped you to bear the pain?
5. In the midst of grieving, how do you care for your physical, emotional, and spiritual self?
6. Name a recent experience of "meeting God" in church.
7. All life ends in death. Do you feel God is more concerned with how we live, or what we die from?
8. Has inner stress ever caused you physical illness?
9. How do you react to the "silences" of God?
10. What does the Bible story say to you about God's love for any ill child?

Chapter 7

The Thorns of My Rose

*T*he month of February found Jeff feeling awfully bad. I wasn't doing too well myself. One of the deacons called and told me that the pastor needed me to do some typing before our meeting that night. With him not knowing what I was going through, I decided to go and help. We couldn't find the keys to the computer room and some changes needed to be made for that Sunday's bulletin. Since it was already late in the afternoon, I felt it would be easier for me to make the changes at my own downtown office. I called home to check on Daddy, and Jeff said he wanted to ride with me.

One of my coworkers, a computer expert, stopped by the office and helped me complete the necessary changes. Jeff got sick at the office and I had to take him back home. When I delivered the bulletins to the church, the dinner meeting was over. No one had thought to save any food for me.

When I arrived home, Jeff informed me that there was no hot water. What else? I was so tired, but sleep would not come. Around midnight, Jeff's friend called to say that a tire had blown out on the car and he had neither jack nor money. Jeff was so worried about his car that I called AAA. The problems seemed to just keep on coming. The phone rang again, around 1:30 A.M., and it was my sister. She said that she had been praying for me and felt I needed to know it. She assured me that God was with me, even though I couldn't pray. She worked hard to convince me that the saints everywhere were carrying me to God in prayer. I had thought my inward screams were silent. My sister had heard them.

Sunday I couldn't move. I prayed for strength to make it to the 6:00 P.M.service, knowing I needed to be there. When Jeff decided to attend the 11:00 A.M. worship, I went with him. The deacons surrounded my son and prayed for him. When we got home, the water was hot! Then my boss called and told me to take some time off and rest. Thank God for the little blessings.

The next day I took Jeff for another CAT scan. He stopped at the desk and asked the nurse to find a doctor for me. The doctor lanced the boil on my waistline and gave me some antibiotics for my cold. Of course she reprimanded me for not seeing her sooner.

When we came home, a cousin called Jeff and told him that he was being punished by God. I just could not believe it. How can people be so cruel? I told Jeff that there was only one Judge and his cousin was not it! We both cried. Then Jeff told me that we had to talk because he was going to die and there were things he wanted to tell me. I told him that I didn't want to hear it. He begged me to listen. I couldn't face a final separation from my very own flesh and blood. Surprisingly, we both got a good night's sleep.

The next morning, Daddy insisted that I go to the bank and cash his check before I went to work. When I brought his money home the nurse called and told me Jeff would have to come back to the hospital for another test immediately. I called Jeff to make arrangements to get him to the hospital, but a friend took him. My daughter went with me and one of our associate pastors met us there. The doctor explained that Jeff had fluid on his heart and surgery was imminent. They took him and removed one and a half gallons of fluid from around his heart. He was in much pain and extremely weak. But the nurse would not allow me to remain with him. He needed to be quiet and to rest. Wanting to run away, die, do anything to stop this torture, I waited until he went to sleep, then went home.

I awoke with tears streaming down my face. I had cried myself to sleep. I wish there were adequate words to describe how I felt. How can you summarize a sense of your soul being severed? My only thought was to get to Jeff. He was in intensive care and had no phone.

Daddy wanted me to bring him some ice cream from the freezer before I left for the hospital. When I stepped into two feet of water, I panicked. It was warm and I knew that the hot water heater was the culprit, but I couldn't think of who to call. I tried to find a plumber. I screamed. I cried. I was hysterical. All I wanted to do was get to Jeff. It finally dawned on me that Jeff's frat brother was a plumber and I called him. He told me to calm down, turn off all the water, tell my father he was coming, and go to the hospital.

Jeff was looking and feeling better when I arrived. When I got back home, all of the water was gone, the pipe on the hot water tank replaced, the sump pump was new, and I never got a bill. It's true that God is good. I am so thankful for all of my brothers and sisters in Christ who stood by me and helped in so many ways. I wish they could be named, one by one. They know who they are. I slept that night.

Saturday came and Jeff wanted to talk about making plans for his death. I couldn't talk about it. I rationalized that God would not put me through that. I was going to die before Jeff. That was the way life was supposed to work. When they moved him out of intensive care, he complained about the pain. The nurse said she couldn't give him any more morphine. He became more depressed as the pain continued and refused food. He began to talk about being tired of this horrible merry-go-round. I reminded him of the song he had once dedicated to me: "I feel like going on. I feel like going on. Though trials come on every hand, I feel like going on!"

At 5:30 A.M. he called to tell me he was feeling better and wanted to come home. I went to work early so I could pick him up that afternoon. I called around 2:00 P.M. to see if Jeff needed anything and the doctor was there. He had told Jeff that he would have to quit work, move back home, and get his business in order. My legs were wooden as I tried to make it to my car. I cried. When I got to the hospital lot, I couldn't get out of the car. I laid my head on the steering wheel and yelled. When I finally got to Jeff's room and he was crying, I cried some more.

My daughter and Doris came to visit and Jeff wanted to talk about his funeral, the worship service, and what to do with his belongings. I was too drained. I refused to think about it. They followed me home and my daughter came in to talk for a while. Jeff called, crying hysterically, wanting me to make a three-way call to his siblings in California. I prayed that God would calm him down so that he could get some rest. I couldn't call them until 10:00 P.M. Chicago time, and when I called him back, he was asleep.

The thought of moving Jeff's furniture out of his apartment was overwhelming. I didn't know where I would get the strength or the energy. But I was confident that God would provide what I needed and would work it out when necessary. The next day I brought Jeff to my house and he cried all day. His friend came to take him for a ride. He was weak, and it was cold, but he was gone for about three hours. I slept. He was more calm when he returned and I fixed him dinner.

I could not look at Jeff without crying. I hated seeing

him suffer. He was in pain and very afraid. I was terrified and fearful as well. I prayed again for added strength. I didn't know how I could make it through this ordeal. I asked God to dry my eyes and to give Jeff relief from the pain. That night I dreamed that I was in the airport to meet my oldest son. I heard someone calling us, and when I turned around, I saw a man, but could not see a face. It was like a shadow. When I turned back to look at my son, he was a shadow also. "God, what does this mean?" My days of denial were over.

My father called me at work the next day to tell me that Jeff was crying constantly. He had made an appointment to talk with our pastor. His younger sister had become his sounding board. He called her at all times of the day or night. In reflective review of our life during this time, Jeff taught me what faith and courage were all about. That night two members of our congregation came over at his request. I heard a song coming from his bedroom. "There is not a friend, like the lowly Jesus. No, not one. No, not one. No one can heal all my heart's diseases. No, not one. Oh, no, not one!" Later I discovered that Jeff was planning his funeral with them.

Jeff talked with our pastor and seemed more at ease. I surely had not talked to him. I thought I could depend solely on God. I didn't know how to turn to anyone else for help. Today I am especially thankful for church members who reached out to us. Through them God has shown me that every time I felt like I couldn't make it another day, love was there to surround me. In the midst of sadness and grief, I experienced love.

The next EKG and X-ray revealed that Jeff's heartbeat was erratic, but his lungs were clear. We stopped to have dinner out, but he didn't have an appetite. At 10:00 P.M. he took a sleeping pill and went to bed. He was up at midnight, unable to sleep. I got up, fixed him soup, and it made him sick. He was complaining about everything. He sounded like dear old Dad. The house was cold, the crackers were stale, and on and on. I took some money from one of his friends and bought him an electric blanket. He was very sick and getting more and more depressed.

That Sunday we went to the 11:00 A.M. worship. I cried through the entire service. Church is a good place to cry—people think you've been touched by the Holy Spirit. Most of them can't tell when you've been affected by a broken spirit. When we got home, Jeff was so weak it was difficult to get him into bed. The next day we went to see a cancer specialist for his first chemo treatment. The doctor was very compassionate and gave Jeff some stronger pain pills. The chemotherapy did not allow him to sleep that night.

I didn't get any sleep either, but I went to work. It was the first time I had worked a full day in weeks. Thank God for an understanding boss. The next day Jeff did go to work all day. He felt fine in the morning and got sick in the afternoon. I suggested that he only work half-days until he got stronger. I don't know how he went at all. I'm sure that the stares and the whispers hurt him terribly, because they hurt me. He was willing to endure them.

It was way past time for me to talk to my pastor. The pastoral counseling helped me tremendously, for Pastor helped me face Jeff's death. I didn't talk much; I listened and I cried. It was difficult to come out of my denial. I knew the facts. Still I wanted to run and to keep on running. Jeff had been trying to talk to me for so long. I didn't want to face this reality.

We went to worship together the next day. Jeff carried his choir robe, but was too weak to sing. He sat with his sister and slept through most of the service. His sister took him to his apartment and I called later to see how he felt.

He had just taken a sleeping pill and asked me to pray for him. I assured him that he was in my prayers constantly. I urged him to continue with his own prayers.

Jeff's car would not start the next morning. He wanted to go to work but was too weak to take public transportation. Doris took me to pick him up and I finally told her the truth. She had guessed, but never asked me any questions. Jeff was so feeble he could barely walk. I tried to talk him into staying home, but he was determined to go work. He only stayed for three hours and I sent a cab to pick him up. That evening he cried as he talked about how he wished he could work all day and not get sick and have to come home. I didn't say a word. I just prayed.

At 2:00 A.M. Jeff woke me. He had dreamed he was well and his body was completely restored. He felt this was a sign that God was going to heal him. I prayed that his dream would come true. That day, February 25, was the sixth anniversary of his father's death. I was glad my husband was not alive. He would not have accepted Jeff's lifestyle, his illness, or my caring for him. It would have been an impossible situation. As tired as I was, with so little help, I was glad he was not here to cause me and Jeff additional anguish.

We had to go see the cancer specialist and Jeff's regular doctor. We didn't get home until 7:00 P.M. Daddy was saying that his gums were sore and he couldn't eat. When I thought about him, I realized that he was eighty-six and had all sorts of health problems. Every time I took Jeff to the doctors, it seemed as if I needed to take Daddy too. My feet were so sore, I could hardly walk. This was a sure sign of how tired I was. I took one of Jeff's pain pills and went to bed. My son called and I couldn't talk. My uncle called to tell me my aunt had been admitted to the hospital. "How much more, Lord?"

When I awoke, I felt like a cloud of gloom was hanging over my head. I wished I could laugh. I wished I could pray. My energy and my motivation were gone. "God, what is this life all about?" Jeff had to go for chemo and he seemed to be feeling better. But when we got home Daddy accused Jeff of stealing all of his clothes. It was all in his mind.

February 28, 1992, Jeff took a ninety-day leave of absence from his job. He asked me again to help him commit suicide. I knew how much he loved his work and was scared that he had given up. I felt whipped and beaten. Even while trying to encourage him to believe God's Word and to hold on, I felt my own grasp on life slipping away. I just wanted a way out. "It's too much, Lord." My sister and I talked, and she asked me where my faith was. I wanted to know too. I didn't know if I had any left. She calmed me down as always. I prayed and gave God thanks for her being in my life.

Jeff's leave of absence brought me face to face with the issue of closing down his dream apartment. I couldn't pay the nine hundred dollars monthly rent. His car was not running and his friend was not working. I was sad, overwhelmed, and felt like the bottom was dropping out of my life. I felt very alone and was growing more and more bitter by the day. I just wanted to stay in bed. I tried to do my morning devotions, but couldn't keep my mind on them. All I could pray was, "Lord, you know."

Jeff came over the next morning and fixed breakfast for himself and Daddy. I prepared to go to work. He told me that I looked tired and asked me to promise him that I would get some rest. This reminded me of the day my husband died, for he had said the same words to me. This upset me, but I thought it sweet that with all of his problems, he was worried about me. I gave God thanks for every morning that I could see and talk with my son. I could hardly wait for him to call me, it was such a pleasure to hear his voice.

It was Ash Wednesday, the beginning of Lent. We are each called to journey with Jesus to Calvary. I never knew his distress before. I was never this close to his grief before. I could not comprehend the meaning of his death and dying before. Now I clearly understood. It was God's grace that allowed me to be consumed by Jeff and Daddy's illnesses, their demands, and a tiredness that I could not imagine being alleviated anytime soon. Yet I worked every day and did whatever I had to do.

Jeff wanted to go to church for the noon worship. My neighbor took him. I went to work early and skipped the services so that I could take him to the doctor. This was the first time I could remember not being at the Ash Wednesday worship. But Jeff was there. He testified and asked the church to pray for me. One of the deacons had embraced him as they prayed for him. I didn't find out until a year and a half later who she was, although Jeff tried to describe her to me. I gave God thanks for those who were loving to my child.

Finally I was forced to face the truth that Jeff was on his final journey back to God. It was Lent.

Reflections

1. Have you experienced a personal season of Lent in your life?
2. Have you ever had a period when you could not pray?
3. What do you think about emotional distress causing physical illness?
4. What do you think you would feel like if your soul were "severed"?

5. Could you help a loved one make funeral plans? How would you feel?

6. What purpose could this have for the dying person? for you?

7. Are there any "good" reasons for this mother's and son's many tears?

8. Is the denial of death Christian? healthy?

9. Does your pastor(s) provide counseling for families touched by AIDS?

10. Is your church a good place to cry?

Chapter   8

His Petals Fall

Jeff had one of his fraternity brothers come and install a vanity in my bathroom as a surprise. Then he asked whether he had made a mistake by taking a leave of absence from his job. His car was not running again. When he got to my house he discovered the new vanity leaking water. The filter on the faucet in the kitchen sink was stopped up and the water trickled, like the tears that ran constantly down Jeff's face. All I wanted was for Jeff to stop crying. "I can do all things through Christ who strengthens me," I affirmed.

My deacons group met and I confessed to a state of exhaustion. They prayed for me and we went to breakfast after our meeting. How I needed a haircut, but couldn't see wasting time on myself. I had to go back to the clinic and pick up some papers for Jeff's job. Then Doris called to tell me that a truck had hit her car and never stopped. She had always been there for me and I didn't even know how to console her.

Jeff had gone to his apartment and taken a ride with his friend. He called upset. While they were out, he had gotten ill. He asked his friend to go into the store and get something for him. His friend refused. I felt hate boiling up inside me. How could he mistreat Jeff at a time like this? That incident must have triggered Jeff's thinking, for he called friends all over the country and came to my house and waited for their return calls. He told me that he wanted to tell them each goodbye. I stretched out prostrate on the floor weeping and wailing in agony.

The intensity, the duration, and the drain of my grief were not familiar to me. The loss of my mother and my husband were painful processes. I thought I had grieved for them. But nothing could have prepared me for this. Many losses or mini-deaths had occurred in the course of my life, so I knew that grief was not just a part of dying but a way of living. Grief must be lived through, endured, and walked with. This must be what David meant when he wrote, "Though I walk through the valley of the shadow of death." Knowledge did not lessen the force of my grief.

As a mother, I had given up Jeff once before to birth. Jeff had been part of me, growing and existing inside of me for nine full months. We knew each other intimately for we were one. There is no greater bond than the one between a mother and her child. We had been attached, but then forced to separate in order for him to be whole. It had been excruciating to deliver him. Giving him up to be born into eternity was no less agonizing. I honored him as God's creation, my gift. Attachment and loss are equal parts of our lives. You gain and you lose. But I was not ready to surrender Jeff to God.

Grief is one of the many rhythms of our lives. It is pervasive and it is persistent. It will not be denied. It is unpredictable, erratic, and sure. Grief can be vicious and hold on until it seems it will never end. You cannot avoid it. You cannot bypass it. You cannot wish it away. Grief is really an "ordinary" element of our lives. It doesn't matter whether you have lost something material, your life's role, or, like me and Jeff, a significant relationship—grief will be present. That's why I believe the songwriter wrote, "What a friend we have in Jesus, all our sins and *griefs* to bear! What a privilege to carry everything to God in prayer!"

Whether you are the one leaving or the one being left,

grief will be encountered. My grief was not identical to the dying process that Jeff was undergoing. Jeff knew that death was the termination point for the life he knew. Grief has no end! Elisabeth Kübler-Ross has listed the stages of dying: denial, anger, bargaining, depression, and acceptance. Although the stages fluctuate and their order changes, dying patients will undergo each one. Even Jesus went through these stages with the exception of denial.

In his humanness Jesus wanted to know from his disciples, "Could you not keep watch for one hour?" (Mark 14:37). That night in the garden, as he struggled and wrestled with the issue of dying, he had asked his friends to accompany him. He had not denied that he was going to die. He was born to die for our sins. He had accepted that responsibility when Adam and Eve sinned in the first garden. Yet he sought community. Even Jesus needed human support in a time of personal crisis. He couldn't handle the "comfortable, fashionable church" where the folks sat sleeping! He refused to allow them to ignore, neglect, and forget that he was facing a turning point in his life. He woke them up and was most likely both hurt and angry for their failure to be present to him in that hour.

Jesus began to bargain with God. "Take this cup from me" (Mark 14:36). The Bible records that despondency, melancholy, and heaviness of heart overtook him. Sounds like depression to me. For Jeff's crying gave indication of similar temperaments ravaging his soul. Finally Jesus accepted his fate: "Yet, not what I will, but what you will" (Mark 14:36). It was time for God's purpose to be accomplished in his life and he surrendered his will.

Jeff surrendered as he called to bid his friends a last farewell. I read somewhere that the term "farewell" was meant to wish those going on a journey that God would assist them on their way and allow them to fare well. Jeff knew he was leaving us, but wanted to assure us that he was in good hands. And he wanted us to "fare well" and not to travel his road of suffering.

With only two hours of sleep I went to worship that Sunday morning. Jeff was too ill to attend. I wanted to stay home with him, but he insisted that I go on to church. I drove to church in a fog. I don't remember the ride. I don't know how I got there. And when I got there I couldn't get comfortable, and was getting ready to go back home when someone told me that Jeff was there. One of his friends had picked him up and he came dressed in the only clothes his thin body could wear—jeans. None of his other clothes fit. My eyes welled with tears as I saw the emaciated frame of my child. At the conclusion of the service I took him home, fixed dinner, and we ate together. Every meal felt like the "last supper."

His friend came to take him to the movies and we had to help him get out of the car when they returned. He took a bath, and asked me to come and pray for him. He said, "Mama, you're a deacon; come and pray for me." We prayed together, thanking God for every minute that we had together. Through it all, we had much for which we were thankful. Jeff was sick, but not bedridden. We recognized that it was God who kept him on his feet.

Jeff was in so much pain that he couldn't sleep that night. I made him some ginger root tea. Nothing else was easing his stomach pain, so it was back to the soothing home remedies. We went to the doctor that day for a blood test and Jeff considered changing doctors. We talked about the myriad of financial problems. The apartment was the last thing he wanted to give up. He loved it so, and I knew that. I didn't want to give it up until he knew for certain that he could no longer keep it.

I always woke up sad, but it seemed that the following morning was the saddest day of all. I was concerned with the emotions of my other children and how they were feeling toward me. They had always felt that I did too much for Jeff. And now I was facing bankruptcy. I prayed that they knew how much I loved each of them. I prayed they could one day understand how much Jeff had need of me during his sickness. Then Doris called to tell me that her car had been totaled. I felt sadder still.

I didn't want to go to work, but work was a blessing in disguise. At work my mind and thoughts were on the job and the concerns there. I yearned to be with Jeff, to spend every possible moment together and to ward off the "enemy." That morning I drove to work alone. Thoughts of suicide began to plague my mind. I wanted, longed for, and sought some relief, some way out. I wouldn't assist Jeff, but I began to think about how I could take my own life.

Jeff called me many times during the day. He wanted me to check on the forms needed for his job. He wanted me to check on the amount of his life insurance. I was not ready. I asked God to forgive me for considering suicide and to give me strength to endure. At home, both Jeff and Daddy needed things from the store. Strength was there for me. One of the deacons called and said she would take Jeff to the doctor the next day. I was thankful.

The new problem was constant hiccups. Jeff went to a breathing specialist who gave him a prescription. I fixed dinner for him and Daddy and went to the drugstore. Somehow I lost Jeff's HMO card. I looked everywhere for it. I had it when I went into the store. I couldn't find it. I ran out of the store crying. I cried all the way home, thinking how careless I was to lose something so important. When I got to the house I was hysterical. Jeff took me in his arms and "mothered" me! "Mama, the card can be replaced. Please don't cry. I can't stand it when you cry." We found the card in the lining of my coat and I went back to get the medicine. I told God, "I can't go on. This is too much for me."

There was no sleep in our house that night. Jeff was sick. When I went to work he was asleep. When I arrived home, both he and Daddy were in bed. He had been calling friends to find someone to take him and get his car. Everybody was busy. I tried to tell him that the car was not important. I begged him to conserve his time and energy. He told me that I didn't care anything about him.

I sat there. He complained that we never talked and he accused me of not spending enough time with him. "Jeff, what do you want to talk about?" Funeral arrangements were on his mind. This was to be the time when he told me what to do with his belongings, what was to be given to his friend and what I was to keep. He told me that he wanted me to have his television and microwave. He was talking like he was going on a trip and making simple plans. I still just sat there.

He had already contacted a friend in Detroit and asked him to direct "Beams of Heaven" during the worship. He told me about the other songs he had selected and who was to sing. He had selected the funeral home. He told me that I wouldn't have to do anything but make arrangements with the church. I sat there praying, "Lord, help me! I'm not made of stone. I can't stand this!"

After work the next day, I walked in to discover that Jeff had terrible diarrhea. I stripped his bed and washed the sheets. He wanted me to take him and his friend to Des Plaines to pick up his car. I took them. They went back to his apartment. Jeff called and I was in the shower. Daddy told me to call him back. Every time he called, I panicked. With wariness, I returned his call. "Mama, I feel so good. I can't believe it. I'm getting well." I gave thanks for being allowed to hear these words. I didn't think they would ever come out of his mouth again. He was so frail that he could hardly move around. And God was providing me with strength daily.

Sunday, March 15, 1992, Jeff waited for his friend to pick him up for the 11:00 A.M. worship. I attended at 8:00 A.M. Returning home, Jeff was in bed, feeling awful because his friend did not pick him up. How I wished I had stayed home to take him to church. This was his last opportunity for public worship, and somehow he knew it. He asked me to buy a tape of the worship. I promised to take him to the men's chorus concert, but he was too sick to attend. He tried to eat dinner, but nothing would stay on his stomach.

One of the members from the choir came by to show Jeff the new robes. He was so excited. He wasn't getting many visitors by this time. He missed going to work, choir practice, and his other activities, so he was glad to see this friend from church. This faithful friend never failed to come by, and even brought money to help meet Jeff's needs. I hope that someday he will be repaid for all of his many deeds of kindness. How I give God thanks for him.

That night Jeff and I finally talked about giving up his apartment. He said that he wasn't sad about it and realized that something needed to be done. Where was I to get the inner strength to move his belongings and store them? How was I going to steal the time and yet be available when Jeff needed me? I went back to night worship, seeking answers. One of our associates preached, "Pray. Then live!" God knew I was trying.

I awoke later than usual the next morning and went in to see about Jeff. He said that he had been sick all night and tried to get my attention. I beat up on myself. "Why didn't I hear him? Why wasn't I there when he needed me?" He took a pain pill and went to sleep. I went to work. Jeff called and asked me to get the doctor to prescribe something for vomiting and diarrhea. Before lunch Jeff called and said he needed to go to the emergency room.

We got there at 1:11 P.M. and they didn't see Jeff until 6:00 P.M. By then he was completely dehydrated and had to have fluids intravenously. They took blood samples and gave him another prescription for medicine that had made him sick before. He told me not to have it filled. I took him home at 10:00 P.M., and he decided we would call his doctor in the morning. I thought about all the many physicians we had seen. All were specialists in their field and gave their best to every patient. I can't say enough good things about them. But Jeff was so weak and extremely tired. They stuck him so many times, in so many different places, just trying to find a vein. I wanted them to stop hurting him. Jeff never complained.

Tuesday I woke up with the familiar tears running down my face. "Lord, I can't stop these tears. Only you can wipe the tears from my eyes." My uncle called to inquire about me and Jeff. I couldn't stop crying. How many times have I said this? I cried at the polling place and was crying at the grocery store when I met two of the deacons from my church. They helped me to find the things I needed, and one gave me information about a home care provider for Daddy.

Jeff called me before I left work and talked about the increasing pain. He was asleep when I got home, so I called his doctor, who told me to take him back to the hospital. They spent hours stabilizing Jeff; his temperature and pulse rate were high and he was dehydrated. It took them hours to find him a room. He stayed in the emergency room for twelve hours. He was weary and so was I. They placed him in a temporary room and Jeff begged me to go home and get some rest. I just could not leave him. Around 1:30 A.M. he fell asleep and I went home to call my sister. For I had told God that my endurance was almost over and my nerves were shot. All I could ask was why. Whether "why" is surrender, acceptance, or resignation, I'm unclear. My rose had wilted. Its petals were falling fast. I could not slow its dying process any longer.

Reflections

1. How does "depression" look? act?
2. Is it possible that Jesus suffered depression?
3. Is all grief the same?
4. What are the losses that have caused you grief recently?
5. If grief is so "common and ordinary," why does it hit us so hard?
6. Can you begin to imagine the grief of the AIDS population? Death is a constant presence.
7. Is it as difficult to say "hello" to new situations as it is to say goodbye to familiar ones (new babies, new jobs, retirement, etc.)?
8. Have you ever played "Let's Make a Deal" with God?
9. How did you move to acceptance of your situation? Or did you?
10. What is there for AIDS sufferers or their families to pray about when death is certain?

Chapter 9

It Is Finished!

I woke up crying. By now it was no surprise. I wondered if I would ever stop. What would happen when the tears ceased to flow? Crying, I called my daughter in California. She could tell that I was crazed from lack of sleep. She told me she was flying home the next day. I went to work and stayed as long as possible. I needed rest. When we talked on the phone, Jeff told me to go home rather than to the hospital. The arrangements were for his sister in Chicago to stay with him that evening.

When I got home, Daddy told me to call Jeff immediately. Jeff was hysterical, having talked to his doctor. I called and found my daughter at the beauty shop. She left to come and pick me up. The doctor met us in Jeff's room. The news was grim. He suggested that I put Jeff in a nursing home. There was nothing else they could do for him. My legs buckled. I pleaded with God for help and strength.

The next morning, crying, I tried to read the Scriptures and do my daily devotions. I didn't know what to do or where to turn. I could not read. I could not pray. I called one of the deacons, who prayed for us. Then I called Jeff and learned he had slept well and was feeling pretty good. I promised to see him after work. Doris picked me up and talked all the way downtown, trying to ease my mind. I couldn't hear her.

My oldest daughter arrived from California around 2:00 P.M. We went to the hospital together. Jeff was so happy to see her, all of us just cried together. She told me that she had no clue that Jeff's illness was so severe. She asked why I hadn't told her. I gave her no answer. We just held each other, standing by Jeff's bed.

The doctor came in and told us that Jeff's liver was failing and his body was riddled with cancer. Jeff could no longer eat and had relentless nausea and diarrhea. Then the doctor said that Jeff would need twenty-four-hour care and would arrange for him to enter a nursing home. I pleaded with the doctor to send Jeff back home to me. I could take care of him. I wanted to take care of him. He was my child, I ought to take care of him. Both the doctor and my daughter replied, "No!"

We told Jeff what the doctor had said. Jeff consented to the nursing home with one condition. I would have to promise him that no one but family would know where he was. I talked openly to God and declared that Jeff could not go into a nursing home. A hospice, home nursing, or something else might work. I could not take the nursing home option. A social worker came to talk about the facility they wanted to send Jeff to, but I wasn't listening. I was still talking to God.

We left the hospital around 5:00 P.M., for my daughter had been up all night. My sister called me and prayed for me before I went to bed. I called Jeff, who said he was feeling all right, even though he was breathing heavily. I prayed and asked God to give my child some rest.

I awoke depressed and exhausted; it took great effort for me to get out of bed. I felt actual pain around my heart. My daughter insisted that we go to see the nursing home. It was nice and clean. Yet I knew in my heart that this would be my only visit there. Heaven was being bombarded with my fervent prayers. Jeff was not going there.

Jeff was quiet when we arrived at his room. He had eaten both breakfast and lunch. The vomiting and diarrhea had stopped. "Thanks be unto God." As I straightened out his linens, I noticed that his legs were swollen. When the nurse was notified, she informed the doctor. Radiation treatments were scheduled for the next two weeks on a daily basis. They were trying to slow down the rate of the cancer's rapid spread.

Jeff went through the first radiation treatment and it made him deathly sick. He couldn't eat and began vomiting again. He asked me to call the desk and get someone to do a living will and power of attorney for him. I told him we would do it the next day. He demanded it be done then. They brought the papers to the room and Jeff signed them. Then he told us that he did not want any lifesaving interventions because he was tired.

Of course I don't remember the drive home. I went straight to bed. Maybe sleep would erase the ache in my heart. With a start, 3:00 A.M. found me sitting up in bed. I remembered that I had not called to wish Jeff a good night. I prayed that he would not think I didn't care. At 3:30 A.M. I was up washing my hair, letting the soapy water mingle with my tears. My daughter got up with the same admonition: "You need rest." I didn't want rest. I didn't care about me. I had ceased to exist. Jeff was my only concern.

It was time to share this news with my brother and his wife. They didn't know he was ill or in the hospital. As I told my sister-in-law, she scolded me for not telling them sooner. I tried to get her to understand that not knowing how she felt about homosexuals, HIV, or AIDS prevented me from telling her. I had done everything possible to prevent Jeff from further hurt. She came to visit Jeff that day.

One of my peers on the board of deacons came to pick me up for a prayer breakfast that had completely slipped my mind. Needing prayer, off we went, and then she dropped me off at the hospital. Jeff was very sick, begging for water and throwing up whenever he tried to drink it. My oldest daughter was with him, trying to help in any way she could. The nurse asked us not to give him anything because the vomiting was wearing him out.

Jeff called me later that evening saying they wanted to give him another test. His endurance had snapped. There was no reasoning with him. He hung up on me and the nurse called and asked me to come back to the hospital and try to calm him down. The weather was snowy and icy. I could barely see. My neighbor was kind enough to chauffeur my daughter and me twice that day. Jeff was insistent that he was tired of needles, tired of tests, and tired of taking medicine. The tests were postponed.

Come Sunday I was numb. I can't describe my feelings. I didn't go to church. My daughters and I decided we needed to talk and arrange a schedule where one of us would be with Jeff on a twenty-four-hour basis. At 11:00 A.M. when we arrived, Jeff was sleeping. The nurse said that he had not slept all night, so we allowed him to rest. He was having vomiting spells and was slightly incoherent. He began having strange dreams. He dreamed about his aunt and told me about it. He had not mentioned her for over a year. He said that he had felt they did not want him around. So he had banished them from his mind. He didn't know that I had called her and asked her forgiveness for not trusting her enough to tell her the truth.

The room began to fill with visitors from the church and his friends from the choir. I especially remember one of the choir members who was having difficulty walking herself. She came just to hold and hug Jeff. My friend Doris came. She could not stay. Jeff's suffering was overwhelming. When he fell asleep, we went home.

Jeff called later to tell me that his friend was coming over to my house. He instructed me to give him the rent for the apartment and money for the phone bill. He came by my house and I told him very politely that Jeff no longer needed an apartment or a phone. And since only Jeff's needs were of concern to me, his days of living off of extended hospitality were over. It was a good feeling to finally tell his friend just what I thought of him. I could not believe that as sick as Jeff was, he had the audacity to ask him for money.

The strength to say no to Jeff's friend assured me that God was indeed preparing me for what was to follow. I knew then that I had something within me with which to face whatever was coming my way.

That Monday I woke up praying. The tears had ceased! My daughter got up and informed me that she was going to move Jeff's belongings out of the apartment right then. I told her that it was impossible. We had no truck, no one to help, no boxes for packing, and nowhere to store five rooms of furniture. She got on the phone and called Jeff's friend who worked for a rental car agency, called her brother-in-law, and called another friend. They went to Jeff's apartment while my granddaughter was "on duty" with Jeff that day.

It was payday and I had to go to work. My granddaughter called to inform me that Jeff had pneumonia again. He was able to talk with me by phone and agreed to take the test, but reminded me of how tired he was. He told me that my granddaughter had been there all day long, by his side, holding his hand, providing comfort. "Mama, she's a real trooper," he said. After work I went to the hospital to allow her to go home.

They gave Jeff a CAT scan and put him on full oxygen. When he was brought back to the room, his friend and I were both there. He began to tell Jeff that I had talked to the manager at the apartment and that plans were underway to move his belongings. The phone rang and it was my daughter saying the truck was loaded and they were on their way to my house. I had thought it was impossible. "With God, all things are possible."

It was my pleasure to tell Jeff's friend that all of his possessions had been left in the apartment and that he was responsible for moving them out. He told Jeff he had to leave right away. When Jeff inquired as to why, he did not respond. I gave God the thanks for allowing my daughter to do what I could not. They brought Jeff's earthly goods and stored them in my basement, with the exception of the television and the microwave he wanted me to have.

Jeff and I were left alone. He asked me to read Psalm 103 and to pray for him:

> Bless the Lord, O my soul,
>   and all that is within me,
>   bless his holy name.
> Bless the Lord, O my soul,
>   and do not forget all his benefits—
> who forgives all your iniquity,
>   who heals all of your diseases,
> who redeems your life from the Pit,
>   who crowns you with steadfast love and mercy,
> who satisfies you with good as long as you live
>   so that your youth is renewed like the eagle's.
> (NRSV)

Jeff told me everything he wanted me to do. He told me what he had asked others to do when he went home to be with God. He told me each song he wanted sung and told me to look in his Bible for the written program. He apologized for not having had the opportunity to select his casket. He had done everything else. He assured me that his sisters would take care of that detail.

Then Jeff said to me, "Mama, I don't want you to have to do anything. You have done so much." He reminded me to keep his television and microwave, and both are in place at my house today. I held Jeff. I hugged Jeff. I told Jeff how very much I loved him. Jeff told me of his love and asked me to forgive him for all he had put me through. Then, typically Jeff's style, he told me that I would be all right. He had already asked the congregation to pray for me.

God's grace is sufficient for me. God gave us the time and the occasion to talk together and to pray our goodbyes. It was God who gave me the fortitude to stand there and to listen to what Jeff had to say without falling apart. Like Mary, the mother of Jesus, I stood there. There were no crowds. We were all alone, enfolded in the love of God and surrendering to this divine will. It was time for me to let him go. It was proper for me to help him be birthed into his new future. I was his mother. We had made this journey together. I could go no further. "It is finished!"

Reflections

1. Who prays for you when you cannot pray for yourself?

2. What is your experience with death and families reuniting to mourn?

3. What do you know about the hospice ministry?

4. Are you familiar with a living will?

5. This mother said that she "ceased to exist" when her child was so ill. Was she codependent, appropriately nurturing, or controlling?

6. Jeff asked his mother to keep another secret. What would you have said?

7. Have the responsibilities of being family caretaker made anyone you know physically ill or emotionally exhausted?

8. Does the reality of Jeff's homosexuality justify the family not being told of his impending death?

9. How do you share "secrets" of this nature?

10. Can making funeral arrangements have a healing effect on the dying?

My Rose Gets New Life

*M*onday, March 24, 1992, I worked a half day while my daughter from California sat with her brother all night. Jeff was too ill even for fluids. The doctor said his kidneys were not functioning and any water would just make his body swell. Jeff begged me for a drink of water and looked at me so sadly when I refused. My heart seemed to shatter. When my youngest daughter arrived, they agreed that I needed to go home and see about Daddy. It was difficult to stay with Jeff and not be able to help him. And it was troublesome for me to leave him.

Jeff put the sheet over his head and got very quiet. I touched him and he replied, "No, Mama. Don't bother me." I waited until he took the sheet off his face. I asked him what he was doing and he told me he was being reconfirmed. I asked him what that meant and he said, "Mama, you're a deacon. You know what confirmation means!" Then he said that someone was calling him and asked me if he should go with the man who was standing in a bright light, holding out his hands. I asked Jeff if he wanted to go. He said, "Not yet."

When my niece called a while later, he told her to come and see him because he would not be here much longer. Jeff had made his peace with God. He had arranged for a celebration of his life. Jeff had selected scriptures and songs that reflected his faith in a new future. His kidneys failed completely. The cancer specialist wanted to give him another test to see how they could relieve the pressure. He was downstairs being tested for two hours. When they brought him back, once again he told me how tired he was and how much pain he was suffering. His regular doctor came to explain what was to be done next. They put in a catheter and Jeff just looked at me with the most unhappy eyes. I told the doctor to stop all treatment.

This was the most difficult decision I had to make in my whole life. There was this struggle within me to have them do all that they could to keep Jeff with me. There was this selfish element within that wanted to hold him close, see him, talk with him, and have him talk to me. Then there was the reality staring me in my face. Jeff had been through enough. He didn't need any more tests. He didn't need another needle. And he would not be forced to take any more medicine. My determination was fixed and my mind was made up. I surrendered Jeff and myself into the care of God. When the girls arrived, I went home to call my sister.

With three hours sleep, I awoke to discover that my tears were accompanying me again. Yet I thanked God for the energy that continued to be supplied. I asked God to stay by my side and to continue holding my hands. When I got back to the hospital, Jeff was restless, like he had been all week. He told me that his sisters were being mean to him, refusing to give him any water to drink. I told him that he could have all of the water that he wanted. I gave him the water and he vomited it right back up. I kept my promise and gave him as much as he wanted.

I sat by his bed and Jeff raised up his arm and asked, "Mama, whose arm is this?" I said, "Jeff, that's your arm." He responded, "No, it isn't. Look how small this arm is, it can't be Jeff's. Jeff is not here." I tried not to comprehend his message to me. He asked me how I was and I replied, "Okay." Jeff said, "Mama, you're not okay. Your hair is not combed." And it wasn't.

His body was swollen tremendously and he was in constant pain. He asked me to call his friend from the choir who had been visiting with him. He asked me to call two additional choir members so he could talk with them. When I told him that I didn't know any of their numbers, he remembered them. I dialed the numbers and got no answers. The three of them walked into his room.

Jeff told me that he wanted to tell me the names of everybody in the room. He named each one I could see and called some who were invisible to me. He called a woman from the choir by name and said she was sitting in the chair. He told me that his favorite high school teacher was walking across the parking lot, coming to see him. I didn't see either of them. He told me that the man was back, with the bright light surrounding him. The man was holding out his hands, beckoning Jeff. He said he was going with the man. I told him I loved him. He said, "I love you too, Mama. Are you sure you're all right?" I assured him that I was. He said, "Go home and get some rest, Mama. I'm all right and I love you."

The doctor said he was going to start a morphine drip so that Jeff would not experience so much pain. He explained that Jeff's body was filling up with water due to kidney failure, and it would soon cover his heart. He was confident that Jeff would sleep peacefully and probably not wake up again. When my baby went to sleep, I went home. I called his brother in California and my sister and told them it was time for them to come home.

At 2:10 A.M. on March 29, 1992, Jeff was born into eternity. Both of his sisters and his niece were with him to witness his tranquil transition. His oldest sister had stayed in the room with him. I could hardly get her to leave. Jeff had always been her baby; it was hard for her to give him up. I made my last trip to the hospital to see Jeff. He was asleep in the arms of Jesus. God got the glory, the honor, and the praise of my lips that night, for Jeff never went to a nursing home. And my child would not suffer ever again.

I went home and went to sleep. Pastor called to comfort me and to ask about funeral arrangements. One of the deacons came to see what needed to be done. I wanted to take a basket of fruit to the nurses who had cared for Jeff. We cried together. They told me that Jeff had already thanked them for everything they had done for him. Jeff had been special to them and they treated him with loving care. They acknowledged never having seen a family stick so close to an AIDS patient before. But they had never met my rose!

All day long I remembered the prayers of people who had sustained me. I recalled the prayers offered in my congregation and the prayers of Jeff's friends from North Carolina to New York. I gave God thanks for making it possible for Jeff to see the other side and for allowing him to cross over in a peaceful sleep. The Women of Worship sang it best on their *Jesus Is the Name* recording:

> All day long, I've been with Jesus.
> All day long, my lips have uttered praise.
>   All day long, my heart, my soul's been
> Lifted, in worship.
> All day long, I have been with him!
> No way could I ever honor
> You enough
> For all that you have done for me.
> So, I will offer up thanksgiving
> From my heart
> And praise, continually! (Carlton J. Fellows)

Monday morning I went into the office to type Jeff's obituary while his sisters and brother made the arrangements at the funeral home. When I got home, a dozen red roses had been delivered to me from Jeff! He had asked one of his friends to send them to me the day after his death. Jeff was alive and alive forevermore!

The discovery was as clear to me as that one made to four women of color who made the journey to the grave of Jesus, prepared to do ministry to a cold, dead corpse. They came to attend to a body that was already wrapped in a winding sheet. It was the last act of devotion they could do for a dead loved one.

Early in the dark, before the first stream of sun streaked across the sky, these women, my sisters, were on their way to the grave. There had been no Hilton or Marriott bed the night before. They had no limo service or escort in this, the most chilling and frightening hour of the day. Yet, in the dusk, women alone, with fragrant spices, washrags, and water pots in their arms, were on their way.

These women were traveling after being in attendance at the crucifixion. With grieving hearts and horrified eyes, they had witnessed the torture of their beloved Jesus. They had been there for hours as he suffered, bled, and died. Then they had been part of a small funeral. They had seen the tomb. They had watched two strong men seal the entrance with a stone at least six feet wide and three feet high. Then they had observed Jewish law and became the official mourners for him. "Call for the wailing women to come; send for the most skillful of them to come quickly and wail over us till our eyes overflow with tears" (Jeremiah 9:17–18). Like me, they could not stop their tears.

Tired, mourning, grieving, and filled with despair, these biblical sisters ask the question of every mother whose heart is breaking as she watches her child die of AIDS. "Who will roll this stone away?" There is a stone that covers our heart. There is a stone that covers our hope. There is a stone that covers our faith. The stone is not a figment of the imagination, but a harsh reality with which we have to deal. But, despite the stone, the sisters are moving toward the grave.

Perplexed by possible difficulties, surrounded by the mysterious unknown, and certain that their own finite capabilities were inadequate, these women pressed forward. The stone was a problem for the future. The tomb would not deter or alter their journey. They projected themselves to the other side. They marched on notwithstanding the question, "Who will roll the stone away?" They never had to seek an answer to this question, for when they arrived at their destination, the stone had been rolled away.

The power of love, the power of this journey, and the power of this story is awesome and compelling. So it amazes me that in the earliest tradition of the church, as recorded by Paul, several decades before Mark ever put his pen to a scroll, these women are neglected as the first witnesses of the resurrection. But it was the women, the sisters, the daughters, the nieces, the aunts, and the mothers who arrived at the grave first. But a dead body was not what they found! The grave was empty! Resurrection had occurred! They found that the Rose of Sharon was alive and his fragrance was stronger than ever before!

Without the testimony of these women, Paul would not have had his story of the resurrection to pass along. Women were the very first ones to know that Jesus was alive, whether their names were in Paul's records or not. And we women continue to do the ministry and the missions assigned by God to our hands, even the pastoral care of journeying through unlit nights to discover flowers that bloom brighter yet.

Reflections

1. Broken hearts and wounded spirits are in great supply in our world. Who is responsible for reaching out and ministering to them?
2. Nursing homes are filled with people who are forgotten. Can we afford to allow people to be discarded and thrown away?

3. What do you think about the man with the bright light beckoning?

4. The decision to stop all interventions is a harsh call for loved ones to make. What do you think this mother's other options were?

5. Why did the mother's tears cease?

6. The nurses were especially kind to Jeff. Have you known of those who neglected terminally ill patients?

7. How did this mother come to "praise" during Jeff's dying process?

8. Are there "mourners" in your local congregation who act out of love and concern for the dying and their families?

9. Has the ministry of the "mourners" been valued in the local church?

10. Why do you believe Paul neglected to mention the pastoral care of the women?

Chapter 11

Celebrating the Life of a Rose

Words fail me as I try to describe Jeff's homegoing celebration. There was such a spirit of celebrating his life and his ministry of help and service. All week long I received phone calls from people I didn't know that Jeff had helped. The worship was unlike any the church had experienced at a funeral before. Jeff had designed and planned the order of service and we followed it. I had asked God to be by my side and to continue to hold my hand. God upheld me and carried me through.

My pastor stood in the center aisle and held my hand that day as I read the following message from Jeff:

Jeff asked me to speak for him today. I told him that I didn't think so. He instructed me, "Mama, write it down and all you have to do is read it." He asked me to tell the choir and the men's chorus how much he loved them and how much he enjoyed singing with them. He wanted to thank everyone for their prayers, visits, cards, and flowers. He told me to thank you for being here today. He even asked me to tell Walter and Shirley thanks for coming to the hospital and inviting him to their wedding. He will be there in spirit.

He asked me to give his friend Donald the twenty dollars he owed on his new robe. Then Don is to give it to someone who needs it, who loves the Lord, and who loves to sing.

He said there were only two things he wanted to do

that were not in God's plan. He wanted to march with the choir into our new sanctuary. And he wanted to go with the choir to Puerto Rico. I know that Jeff will be there.

Well Jeff, I followed your orders and spoke for you today. And Jeff, I am all right. Thank you for the roses.

Jeff, you taught this family that God is good all the time. And I now know the peace that surpasses all understanding. Thank you, God. Love ya, Jeff.

Mama

Everything was perfect. The sermon was a masterful creation by our pastor. The choir sang with a special anointing. The soloists rendered healing ministry to our souls. We worshiped and gave God thanks for the gift of my rose. My entire family was there, sister, brother, children, grandchildren, and great-grandchildren. "A mighty fortress is our God, a bulwark, never failing!"

Chapter 12

The Fragrance Lingers Still

My tears are on every page of this book. It has not been easy to sit down and write the story of the journey I made with my son through the land of HIV/AIDS. For many years I have kept a journal. It has been a way of talking with God, reflecting on my life, and seeing how God has brought me through. Going back and reliving every horrible day of this battle with AIDS was a difficult task. I prayed for strength every time I sat down to write. For I still cannot talk about Jeff without crying, I have not been able to listen to the audiotape of his homegoing worship, and I cannot visit the cemetery. Someday. Sometime in the future my strength will allow me to accomplish these tasks, but not yet.

Jeff had a life before AIDS. He was a loving and outgoing man. You already know his commitment to Christ and the church of the living God and his devotion to the ministry of music. Jeff had many friends and always treated them as brothers and sisters. His world was not closeted and secret, but wide and vast as he gave of himself. He was passionate about his work with young people, and much of this passion was carried out in connection with his beloved fraternity. Jeff's smile would light up a room and his laugh was an enjoyable outburst. You can tell much about a man's character by how he treats his mother. Throughout his short life, my son cared about and for me. He included "Mama" in his circle of connections and trusted me with many of his secrets. His selected gift to me, the flower of love, on every special occasion speaks volumes. And every time I see a rose, I think of my Jeff and I smile.

With all of his attributes, Jeff would not have stood out in a crowd of his peers, for he was involved with friends who complemented him in service projects and ministry. It was his battle with AIDS, the faith he had in God, his confidence in Scripture, and his belief in the power of prayer that made my son outstanding. This work is dedicated to the memory of a great man of God, my son, Jeffery Lynn Bell. He taught me about faith during our journey. He showed me a first-rate courage. He exhibited outstanding character as he attended church until the very last. He modeled love for his family. And he evidenced caring concern for me. It is these admirable qualities, demonstrated in extreme illness, that set Jeff apart and made this book mandatory writing.

I learned how to do caring ministry with others during my care for Jeff. The experience taught me how to reach out to others who are gripped in despair and cannot ask for help. I learned how to do spiritual warfare in this battle for Jeff's life. It is the enemy of our souls who seeks to divide us as family and to set us against those we do not understand. It is evil the way the church can forget, neglect, and not see the lepers of our day. Jesus saw them and ministered to them. And that's reason enough for me. Without my having to encounter HIV/AIDS face to face, my eyes might yet be closed to the great epidemic in the African American community. Sometimes I wish that my eyes had not been opened. But I can see clearly now, and there is much work for us to do.

Life did not settle down and get smoother after Jeff died. My uncle's wife, my beloved aunt, died three months after Jeff, in June 1992. Daddy died three months after her, in September 1992. They say that death always comes in threes.

Nineteen ninety-two was not an easy year, but a span when I truly experienced amazing grace. My faith grew that year, by leaps and bounds. My limits were stretched and I endured. God taught me many lessons and pulled forth gifts from within me that had never been tapped before. Yes, I lost a lot. And I gained a lot in exchange.

It is no secret that I belong to Trinity United Church of Christ in Chicago, Illinois, where the Reverend Dr. Jeremiah Wright is my pastor. I deliberately did not want to mention the name of my church in the previous pages, for it could have been any church anywhere in America. Trinity cannot be singled out as having all the homophobic Christians in America.

Over the years since Jeff's death, I have seen great growth and acceptance in Trinity's congregation toward those afflicted with AIDS. Pastor Wright has been at the forefront of this significant progress. In December of 1993 the newly formed HIV/AIDS ministry was brought before our congregation and blessed by our pastor. More than thirty members joined the ministry team and received twenty hours of training. In September of 1994, when additional training was held, more members joined. For every caring minister in this group, I give God thanks. It is especially meaningful to me that one of Jeff's best friends is now actively involved.

I have experienced spiritual growth and development in my own life and have been able to effectively minister comfort to other mothers as far away as California. Whenever Pastor gets word that one of our members is affected, he dials my number or catches me in the hall. I have gone to the vast AIDS network at Cook County Hospital to take communion to the patients and their families. When I see them crying and depressed, when I see their suffering and loneliness, and when I notice there is no family member present, I can identify with and be a caring presence in their lives. God blessed me with Doris and other good friends who have been there with me and continue to reach out in my times of loneliness. And they do come. It is about giving back some of what I have received that inspires me to minister.

My daughters are working to educate African American people about this disease. For AIDS has no boundaries. AIDS conquers prejudices and crosses ethnic, racial, gender, age, and economic barriers. AIDS is not a gay disease, but a human disease affecting many African American people. If you don't know anyone who has died from AIDS, you will shortly. AIDS touches us all. Every year Trinity holds a candlelight memorial service for those who have died of AIDS. The number of candles increases as we remember their lives and call their names. They live on in our hearts. They teach us how to care.

I know that Jeff's life and death have made an impact on our local congregation. Progress has been made. Because of awareness and new knowledge, families are not as subject to the whispers and shunning that Jeff and I came to know so well. The week before Jeff died, one of the deacons in our congregation came to visit my son. When he found out that Jeff had AIDS, he ran out of the room. So much for pastoral care and Christian love. Some of our HIV/AIDS ministers have the disease themselves. They've become our most valuable assets. I will always remember Gayle, a young black mother. Gayle shared her story, her life, herself with this ministry. She learned much about the disease she had and she taught us much about how to live with it. When Gayle died, a bright light in our ministry team went out.

In December of 1995 we joined with the Balm in Gilead, a resource bank out of New York that sponsors an annual black church day of prayer for the healing of AIDS the first Sunday in March. A not-for-profit secular organization started by Pernessa C. Seele, its mission is to prevent the transmission of HIV/AIDS among African Americans and to support those already infected by mobilizing the religious community to address the issues appropriately and effectively. Seele is a black woman who has done extensive work with the Centers for Disease Control and Prevention in Atlanta, seeking to educate and serve African Americans by mobilizing the most effective voice in our communities, the black church. Trinity holds a concert on Friday night and an all-day workshop on Saturday prior to World AIDS Day focusing on the care of both patient and family. AIDS is running rampant in our communities. Education is needed. I am compelled to spread the word.

My life reminds me of the woman at the well. For John 4:4 tells us that Jesus needed to go through Samaria. There was a foreign woman who had a hole in her soul who needed her cup filled with Living Water. I like the mandate that Jesus followed, "I must go to Samaria!" The Jews treated Samaritans as if they had AIDS. They were the social outcasts of Jewish society. A "good" Jew would walk an extra distance to prevent touching the land of a Samaritan. Yet Jesus deliberately set out for Samaria.

Forty-two verses of dialogue. Jesus and this nameless woman talked for a long period of time. Forty-two verses of conversation. This is the longest of any verbal exchange between Jesus and anyone else, even the disciples. Forty-two verses and they had a theological discourse about renewing, reviving, and receiving the refreshing water that would spring up within; they talked about true worship of God and they spoke of his messiahship, which he had not even revealed to the disciples.

From these forty-two verses, there are three that deal with the woman's inner needs. There are three verses that allow us to see Jesus touch her at her core. In these three verses her hurt is revealed and Jesus offers effective pastoral care.

He does not condemn her, but sets her free from her self-imposed limits to do ministry in his name. This woman leaves her water pot to go running into the city with a message. Her ministry is released. Her compassion is genuine. Her eyes are opened to see the needs of her kin. Her hands reach out to touch those who had avoided her. Her ministry is one of care. Her ministry causes her to become actively involved. "Come and see a man . . ."

The town follows her back to Jesus. The town listens to what she has to say. The town is persuaded that her message is authentic and they go to hear Jesus. Many of them are converted. She becomes the first evangelist to the Gentiles. And it happened because Jesus had a need to go through her town and see about her.

My rose was afflicted with one of the most horrible and devastating diseases this world has ever known. I made a covenant to walk with him all the way. When we began our journey, Jesus had a need to come and see about me. I pray that families who have loved ones dying from AIDS will read this book and come to realize the blessings they are missing by not drinking from the well. Jesus has a need to touch lives. Jesus has a need to make the wounded whole. Jesus has a need to offer salvation and a balm in Gilead.

Because Jesus had a need to come and minister to me and to Jeff, I know without a doubt that the words of Isaiah 43:2 are faithful and true:

> When you pass through the waters, I will be with you; and when you pass through the rivers, they will not sweep over you. When you walk through the fire you will not be burned; the flames will not set you ablaze.

I am a witness that this is true. I have passed through the waters of many tears and I did not drown. I have walked through the fire of HIV/AIDS, and have not been consumed.

For a while I thought I was losing my son. I discovered that the fragrance of my rose is stronger and more fragrant than ever before. May God always bless you and give you a willing heart to stop and smell the roses.

Reflections

1. Why did this particular book interest you?
2. What have you learned about HIV / AIDS from reading this book?
3. What is the most valuable information in this book for you?
4. What will you do with this information?
5. Since nothing happens by "accident," how will what you have learned impact what you do?
6. Are you presently involved in or have you been called to be part of a caring ministry?
7. What spiritual gifts are needed for effective caring ministry?
8. What spiritual gifts do you possess for use in building Christ's realm?
9. What role does remembering life events play in the death and dying process?
10. How does a fragrance become stronger after the flower has wilted?

A Personal Note to Jeff

On Friday, November 12, 1994, I walked into our new sanctuary and sat down on the front pew. I said aloud, "Jeff, I am here!" I know you saw me and rejoiced.

Love ya, Jeff,

Mama

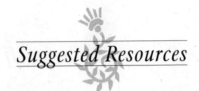

Suggested Resources

AIDS Action Council, 729 Eighth Street SE, Suite 200, Washington DC 20003.

American Foundation for AIDS Research, 5900 Wiltshire Blvd., Los Angeles CA 90036.

Dr. Patrick Dixon, *The Whole Truth about AIDS,* Thomas Nelson, Inc., P.O. Box 141000, Nelson Plaza at Elm Hill Pike, Nashville TN 37214-1000.

Mothers of AIDS Patients, P.O. Box 3132, San Diego CA 92103.

National Council of Churches / AIDS Task Force, 475 Riverside Dr., Room 572, New York NY 10115.

National Leadership Coalition on AIDS, 1150 17th Street NW, Suite 202, Washington DC 20036.

Granger Westberg, *Good Grief,* Augsburg Fortress, 426 S. Fifth St., Box 1209, Minneapolis MN 55440-1209.

Who Will Break the Silence? Liturgical Resources for the Healing of AIDS, The Balm in Gilead, Inc., 130 W. 42nd St., New York NY 10036.